CT
at a Glance

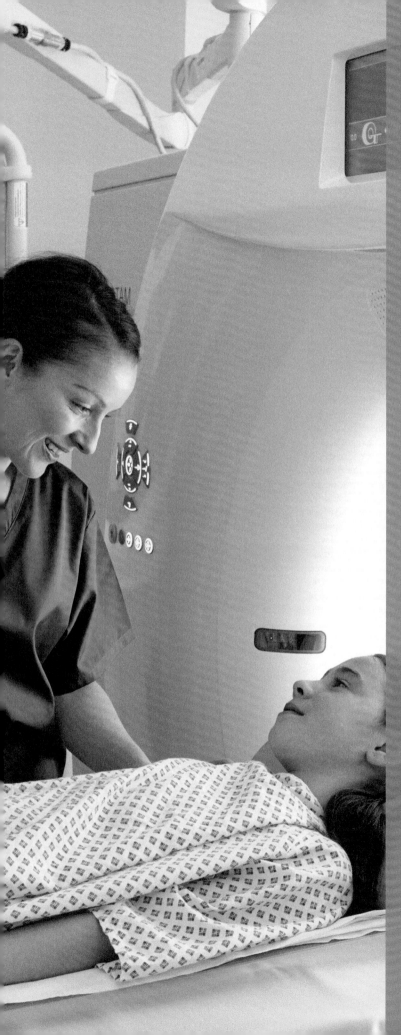

CT
at a Glance

First Edition

Euclid Seeram, PhD, MSc, BSc, FCAMRT
Medical Imaging and Radiation Sciences,
Honorary Senior Lecturer,
Faculty of Health Science,
University of Sydney,
Australia;

Adjunct Associate Professor,
Medicine, Nursing, and Health Sciences,
Monash University,
Australia;

Adjunct Professor,
Faculty of Science,
Charles Sturt University,
Australia;

Adjunct Associate Professor,
Faculty of Health,
University of Canberra,
Australia

WILEY Blackwell

Registered Offices: John Wiley & Sons, Inc., 111 River Street, Hoboken, NJ 07030, USA
John Wiley & Sons Ltd, The Atrium, Southern Gate, Chichester, West Sussex, PO19 8SQ, UK

Editorial Office: 9600 Garsington Road, Oxford, OX4 2DQ, UK

For details of our global editorial offices, customer services, and more information about Wiley products visit us at www.wiley.com.

Wiley also publishes its books in a variety of electronic formats and by print-on-demand. Some content that appears in standard print versions of this book may not be available in other formats.

Library of Congress Cataloging-in-Publication Data

Names: Seeram, Euclid, author.
Title: CT at a glance / Euclid Seeram, PhD., MSc., BSc., FCAMRT.
Description: Hoboken, NJ : John Wiley & Sons, 2017. | Includes index. |
    Identifiers: LCCN 2017025967 (print) | LCCN 2017040984 (ebook) | ISBN
    9781118660881 (pdf) | ISBN 9781118660898 (epub) | ISBN 9781118660904 (pbk.)
Subjects: LCSH: Tomography.
Classification: LCC RC78.7.T6 (ebook) | LCC RC78.7.T6 S3715 2017 (print) |
    DDC 616.07/57—dc23
LC record available at https://lccn.loc.gov/2017025967

Cover image: © Phil Boorman/Gettyimages
Cover design by Wiley

Set in Minion Pro 9.5/11.5 by Aptara

10 9 8 7 6 5 4 3 2 1

This book is dedicated with love and affection to my beautiful, smart, and over-all cute and witty granddaughters

CLAIRE and CHARLOTTE

You bring so much joy and happiness to our lives

Contents

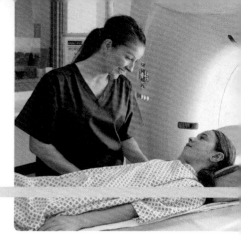

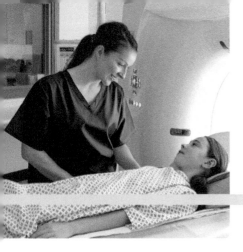

Foreword

Dr Euclid Seeram is a distinguished and rigorous academic who has a proven track record in providing understandable and comprehensive radiological manuscripts. He has decades of experience in the teaching of CT physical principles and medical imaging sciences.

A hallmark of his approach is the ability to convey complex topics in an easy-to-read and manageable way, and this work is no exception. He presents his topics in an organized, progressive, and comprehensive manner so that at the end of each clearly defined chapter, learning objectives are met and the reader comes away with a solid and supported knowledge of specific topics. Euclid has decades of experience in the teaching of CT and medical imaging, and during this time has gained worldwide respect as an educator. Both clinicians and physicists in the field of medical imaging are in agreement with the high level of influence Euclid has on medical imaging education and on the profession as a whole. He is simply a global leader in his field. Euclid's published works have made an impact on radiologic science and technology education, and in particular computed tomography (CT).

This book, *CT at a Glance*, is another means of bringing an understanding of CT to radiographers, radiologic technologists, and others interested in CT physical principles. The technical and clinical developments of CT have continued over recent years and its use in medicine has proven that it is significant and an important diagnostic imaging tool for clinicians to aid in their diagnosis. *CT at a Glance* provides an easy understanding of this complex diagnostic imaging modality.

Euclid must be commended for his continued efforts in making CT and other medical imaging technical knowledge easy to understand by students and clinicians.

Rob Davidson, PhD, MAppSc (MI), BBus, FIR
Professor in Medical Imaging
Head, Discipline of Medical Radiations
University of Canberra
Canberra, Australia

Preface

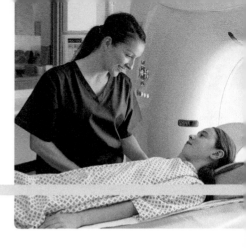

Computed tomography (CT) has experienced significant technological advances ever since its invention in the early 1970s. These advances are meant to improve the scanning speed and reduce the dose to the patient without compromising the diagnostic quality of the image. A few of these significant and important advances include scanners that can image multiple slices in a single breath-hold (multislice CT systems), new detector technologies, automatic exposure control (tube current modulation), automatic voltage selection (X-ray spectra optimization), X-ray beam collimation strategy, iterative reconstruction algorithms that enable scanning at significantly lower doses while maintaining image quality, dual-energy CT scanners that can image the beating heart with excellent detail, and dose optimization strategies, to mention but a few.

The book describes the physical basis for CT and focuses on theory that is essential for practice. Educationally it is pitched at the entry-level for radiographers and radiological technologists, focusing on fundamental physics and technical principles. The main feature of this book is that it provides alternative descriptions of existing knowledge, through the use of multiple illustrations to describe the essential knowledge base for understanding CT physics and instrumentation. Already

various radiography organizations such as the American Society of Radiological Technologists (ASRT) and the Canadian Association of Medical Radiation Technologists (CAMRT) have introduced selected topics in Computed Tomography (CT) for what they label as "entry-to-practice" requirements. The purpose of this text is to meet these requirements, and those of other professional organizations for radiographers and radiological technologists in other parts of the world. This book will serve as a resource for entry-to-practice students in medical imaging technologies such as radiography, nuclear medicine, and radiation therapy. Furthermore, this book can also be used by biomedical engineering technology students studying CT physical principles, CT image quality and quality control as well as radiation protection in CT.

The content and organization are based on 24 chapters ranging from historical perspectives, basic physics concepts, multislice technologies, data acquisition strategies, equipment components, image reconstruction, and image quality considerations to CT dose and dose optimization procedures, and quality control fundamentals.

Read on, learn, and enjoy. *Your patients will benefit from your wisdom.*

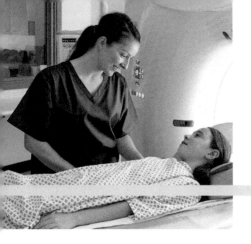

Acknowledgements

A very satisfying task in writing a book of this nature is to acknowledge the help and encouragement of those individuals who believe that such brief notes on a topic that has been described and discussed in volumes is a worthwhile contribution to the computed tomography (CT) literature. I am grateful to several individuals whose time and efforts have contributed tremendously to this work. First I must express sincere gratitude to Dr Godfrey Hounsfield (whose signature is included in the textbook as an illustration in Figure 1.6, and Dr Allan Cormack, who shared the Nobel Prize for Medicine and Physiology for their work in the invention and development of the CT scanner. Secondly, I have learned a good deal of CT physics and instrumentation from seven medical physicists whose published works are invaluable to the CT community. In particular, I am indebted to Professor Willi Kalender, PhD, Institute of Medical Physics in Germany; Dr Jiang Hsieh, PhD, Chief Scientist with General Electric Healthcare; Dr Mahadevappa Mahesh, PhD, Chief Physicist, Johns Hopkins Hospital in Baltimore; Dr Michael McNitt-Gray, PhD, University of California; Dr Cynthia McCollough, PhD, Mayo Clinic; Dr Thomas Flohr, PhD, Siemens Medical Solutions, Germany; and last but not least, Dr John Aldrich, PhD, Vancouver General Hospital, University of British Columbia, whose seminars on radiation dose in CT and other topics have taught me quite a bit.

The content of this book is built around several key principles and concepts of CT that appear to be commonplace in the literature. Examples include physics of CT, technological developments such as those in multislice CT, image reconstruction such as the recent iterative reconstruction algorithms, which all major vendors include with their CT scanners, image quality and dose optimization, and quality control. Furthermore, I must acknowledge the efforts of all the individuals from several CT vendors who have assisted me generously with technical details and images for use in the book. In addition I appreciate the assistance of Magan Stalter of The Phantom Laboratory, Incorporated, Salem, NY, and Pamela Durden of Gammex Inc., Middleton, WI, who have provided the images of QC phantoms for use in the book.

I must also acknowledge the work of the reviewers of this book (listed separately) who offered constructive comments to help improve the quality of the chapters. Their efforts are very much appreciated. The people at John Wiley and Sons, Ltd, in the UK deserve special thanks for their hard work, encouragement, and support of this project. In particular I would like to thank Karen Moore, who realized the value of this project and worked hard to get it through the approval process that led to a contract. Furthermore, I must thank Jennifer Seward for her continued communications with me while writing and responding to reviewers' suggestions. They have both offered sound and good advice in bringing this book to fruition. In addition, I am grateful to Robert Hine and Kathy Syplywczak for their careful and excellent work in shaping the manuscript to its final form.

My family deserves special mention for their love, support, and encouragement while I worked many hours of the day on this manuscript. I appreciate the efforts of my lovely wife, Trish, a warm, caring, and overall special person in my life, and the cutest chaplain I know; to my son David, and daughter-in-law, Priscilla, thanks for your support. This book is dedicated with all my love to my two granddaughters, Claire and Charlotte, beautiful, smart, and witty children

Furthermore, there are two individuals who have always put me on a pedestal: Professor Patrick Brennan, PhD (University of Sydney, Australia), and Professor Rob Davidson, PhD (University of Canberra, Australia). To my good friend and colleague, Anthony Chan, PhD, MSc, PEng, CEng, a Canadian award-winning biomedical engineer, I am grateful for the stimulating and useful discussions of various CT topics. Last, I am also grateful to the thousands of students who have diligently completed my CT Physics course. Thanks for all the challenging and stimulating questions. Keep on learning and enjoy the pages that follow.

Euclid Seeram, PhD, MSc, BSc, FCAMRT
British Columbia, Canada

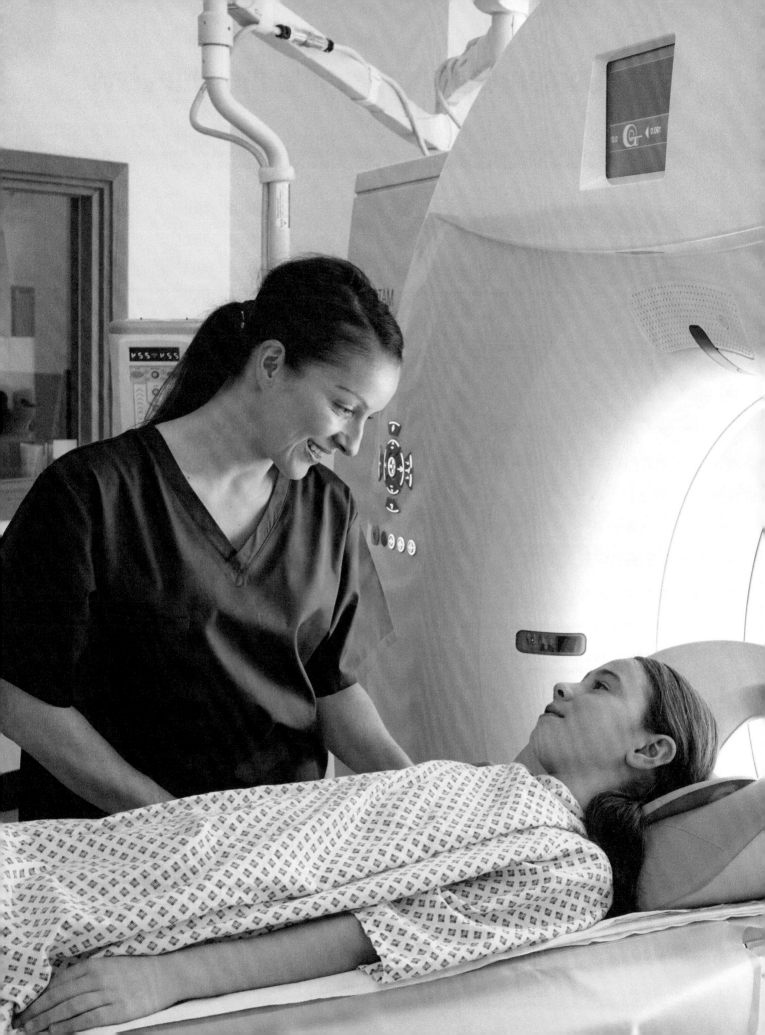

1 Computed tomography: an overview

Figure 1.1 A conspicuous difference between CT and current radiographic imaging is that CT creates and shows cross-sectional and three-dimensional (3D) images from the sectional image data sets; radiographic imaging produces planar images.

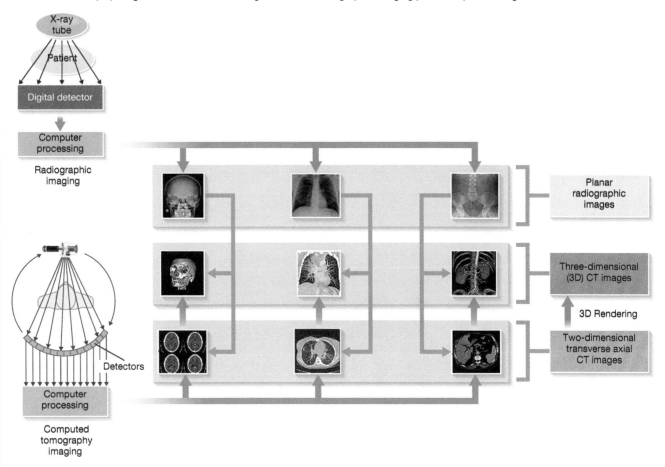

Figure 1.2 The major components of a CT imaging include the CT scanner, the CT computer system, and the operating console.

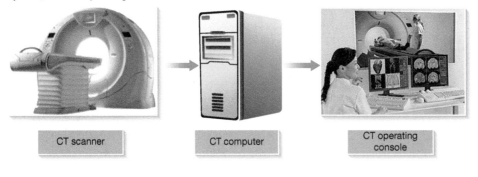

Figure 1.3 The process of CT involves three essential steps: data acquisition, image reconstruction, and image display, storage, and communication.

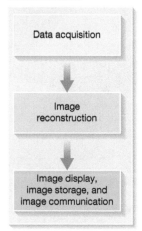

CT at a Glance, First Edition. Euclid Seeram.
© 2018 John Wiley & Sons, Ltd. Published 2018 by John Wiley & Sons, Ltd.

Introduction

A significant and important technological innovation that has now become a popular tool for diagnostic imaging of patients is computed tomography (CT), an imaging technique that was first investigated as early as 1967. Later, in 1971, a prototype CT scanner for imaging the brain was developed by EMI Limited (Electric and Musical Industries [a manufacturer of records and electronics; the Beatles recorded under the EMI label], now Thorn EMI) in Middlesex, UK. This prototype resulted in the first patient being scanned in 1971, and this development earned two pioneers of CT, Godfrey Hounsfield and Allan Cormack, the Nobel Prize in Medicine in 1979.

A striking fundamental difference between CT and current radiographic imaging is clearly illustrated in Figure 1.1. While CT creates and shows cross-sectional and three-dimensional (3D) images from the sectional image data sets, radiographic imaging produces planar images. There are other differences between these two imaging modalities, which will be described in later chapters. One such example is that CT uses much more sensitive electronic detectors, which can show very small differences in tissue attenuation compared to radiographic detectors. This characteristic results in CT providing much better tissue image contrast than radiography, and therefore the observer can see soft tissues much better than with radiography.

Radiographic imaging

The major components of radiographic imaging includes an X-ray tube and generator that provide the appropriate X-rays to image the patient, a detector that captures X-rays transmitted through the patient, a computer processing system, and an image display workstation (Figure 1.1). X-rays transmitted through the patient are converted into digital data for processing by the computer. The image output from the computer is subsequently displayed for viewing and interpretation by an observer. These radiographic images are usually referred to as *planar images*. The problems with these images are (i) superimposition of all structures on the detector (which makes it difficult and sometimes impossible to distinguish a particular detail) and (ii) the qualitative nature of radiographic imaging. The latter simply means that it is difficult to distinguish between a homogeneous object (one tissue type) of non-uniform thickness and a heterogeneous object (bone, soft tissue, and air) of uniform thickness. Finally, the beam used in radiography is an open beam (wide beam) and this creates more scattered rays, which get to the image and essentially destroy the image contrast.

CT imaging

CT overcomes these limitations by removing the superimposition of structures, improving image contrast, and imaging very small differences in tissue contrast.

The major components of a CT imaging are shown in Figure 1.2 and include the CT scanner, the CT computer, and the CT operating console. Furthermore, the process of acquiring images of the patient involves three steps shown in Figure 1.3, data acquisition, image reconstruction, and image display, storage, and communication.

The CT scanner contains the X-ray tube and detectors, which rotate around the patient to collect attenuation data. These data are subsequently sent to the CT computer, which produces images using image reconstruction algorithms (computer programs that build up the image using the attenuation data). Furthermore, CT imaging now creates several 3D image types (Figure 1.1) using what is referred to as 3D rendering algorithms. These image types are intended to enhance diagnostic interpretation. Finally images are displayed for viewing and interpretation, after which they are stored for retrospective analysis, and sent to another location using computer network communications technology. One such popular technology is a Picture Archiving and Communication System (PACS).

As noted earlier, CT produces cross-sectional images of patient anatomy, which are transverse axial sections (Figure 1.4a). These images are referred to as *transverse axial images* (Figure 1.4b). These sections are perpendicular to the long axis of the patient as illustrated in Figure 1.4a.

Figure 1.4 A notable feature of CT is the production of cross-sectional images of patient anatomy called transverse axial sections (a), which are perpendicular to the long axis of the patient. These images are referred to as *transverse axial images* (b).

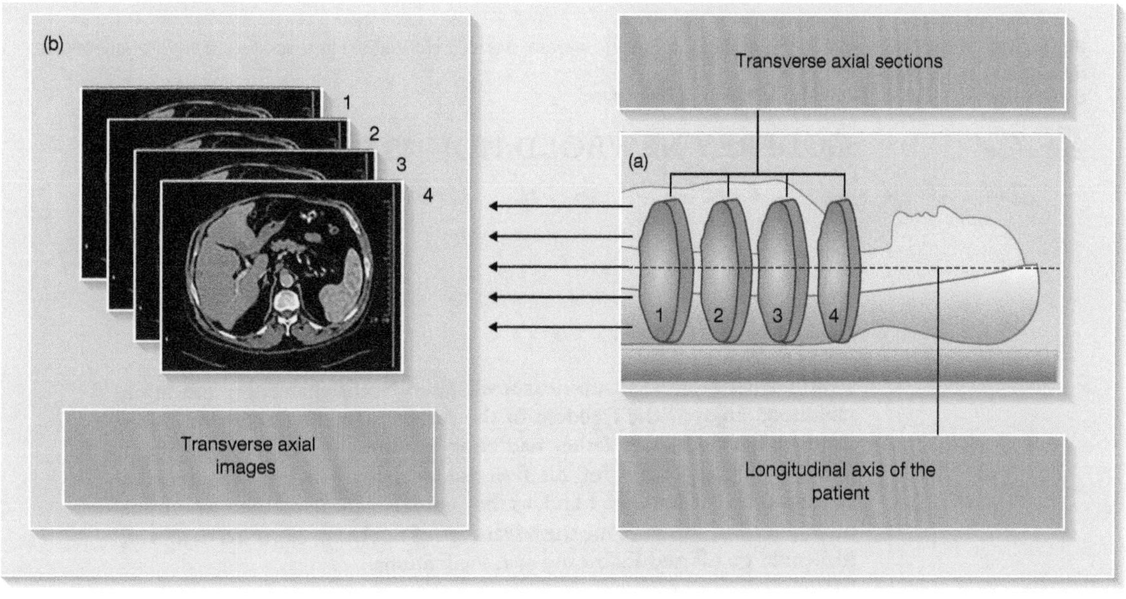

Nobel prize for the invention of the CT scanner

The invention of the CT scanner is credited to two individuals (Godfrey Hounsfield and Alan Cormack) working in two separate countries and who shared the Nobel Prize in Medicine in 1979 for their contributions to the development of the scanner. Photographs and detailed notes of their work are published by the Nobel Foundation (http://www.nobelprize.org). A summary of each of their contributions is shown in Figure 1.5. It is interesting to note the title of their Nobel Lectures. While Hounsfield's lecture is entitled "Computed Medical Imaging," Cormack's lecture is entitled "Early Two-Dimensional Reconstruction and Recent Topics Stemming from It." Both of these pioneers worked out the mathematical solutions to the problem in CT, but Hounsfield developed the first useful clinical CT scanner. Figure 1.6 shows a note sent to the author, Dr Euclid Seeram, from Dr Hounsfield in response to several questions relating to his early work.

Figure 1.5 A summary of each of the contributions of Nobel Prize winners Godfrey Hounsfield and Alan Cormack for their pioneering work in the invention of the CT scanner. Note the title of their Nobel Lectures. While Hounsfield's lecture is entitled "Computed Medical Imaging," Cormack's lecture is entitled "Early Two-Dimensional Reconstruction and Recent Topics Stemming from It."

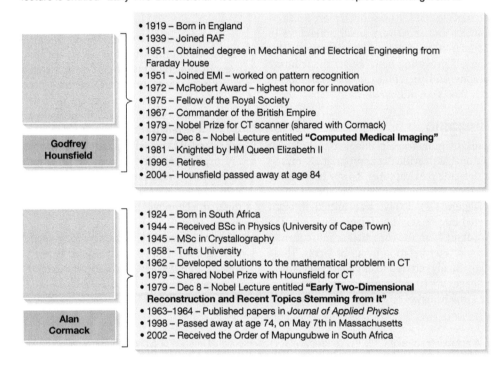

Godfrey Hounsfield

- 1919 – Born in England
- 1939 – Joined RAF
- 1951 – Obtained degree in Mechanical and Electrical Engineering from Faraday House
- 1951 – Joined EMI – worked on pattern recognition
- 1972 – McRobert Award – highest honor for innovation
- 1975 – Fellow of the Royal Society
- 1967 – Commander of the British Empire
- 1979 – Nobel Prize for CT scanner (shared with Cormack)
- 1979 – Dec 8 – Nobel Lecture entitled **"Computed Medical Imaging"**
- 1981 – Knighted by HM Queen Elizabeth II
- 1996 – Retires
- 2004 – Hounsfield passed away at age 84

Alan Cormack

- 1924 – Born in South Africa
- 1944 – Received BSc in Physics (University of Cape Town)
- 1945 – MSc in Crystallography
- 1958 – Tufts University
- 1962 – Developed solutions to the mathematical problem in CT
- 1979 – Shared Nobel Prize with Hounsfield for CT
- 1979 – Dec 8 – Nobel Lecture entitled **"Early Two-Dimensional Reconstruction and Recent Topics Stemming from It"**
- 1963–1964 – Published papers in *Journal of Applied Physics*
- 1998 – Passed away at age 74, on May 7th in Massachusetts
- 2002 – Received the Order of Mapungubwe in South Africa

Figure 1.6 A brief note sent to the author, Dr Euclid Seeram, from Dr Hounsfield in response to several questions relating to his early work.
Source: Copyright 2009 by Saunders, an imprint of Elsevier Inc.

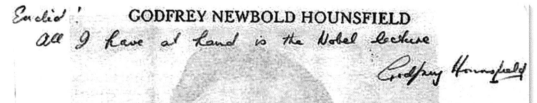

Euclid!
All I have at hand is the Nobel lecture

Godfrey Hounsfield

GODFREY NEWBOLD HOUNSFIELD

I was born and brought up near a village in Nottinghamshire and in my childhood enjoyed the freedom of the rather isolated country life. After the first world war, my father had bought a small farm, which became a marvellous playground for his five children. My two brothers and two sisters were all older than I and, as they naturally pursued their own more adult interests, this gave me the advantage of not being expected to join in, so I could go off and follow my own inclinations.

The technical evolution of CT

CT has experienced a number of significant technical innovations through the years as illustrated in Figure 1.7. In brief CT has evolved from a scanner dedicated to imaging the brain only to single-slice whole-body scanners and multislice scanners, and subsequently to scanners with two X-ray tubes coupled to two sets of detectors. These latter scanners are known as Dual Source CT (DSCT) scanners. Other notable technical innovations include the development of multislice detectors, iterative reconstruction algorithms, virtual reality imaging methods, dose optimization methods, and important quality control test tools and procedures.

These innovations are intended not only to improve image quality and reduce radiation dose, but also to play a role in the care and management of the patient, during CT imaging.

Figure 1.7 Significant technical developments of the CT scanner from Hounsfield's prototype to potential future innovations.

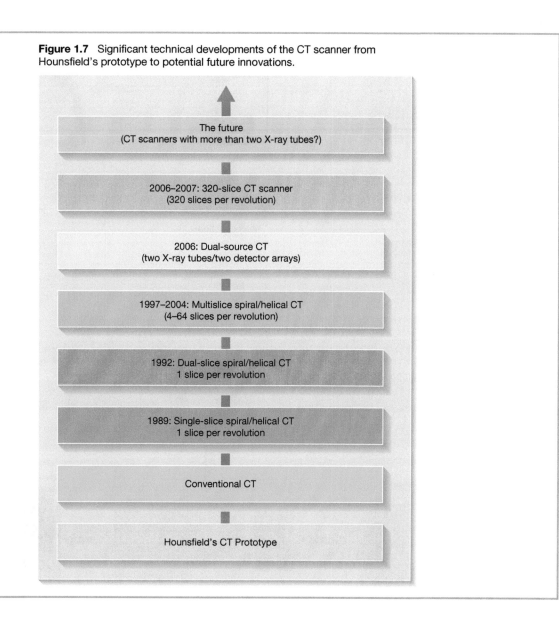

The future
(CT scanners with more than two X-ray tubes?)

2006–2007: 320-slice CT scanner
(320 slices per revolution)

2006: Dual-source CT
(two X-ray tubes/two detector arrays)

1997–2004: Multislice spiral/helical CT
(4–64 slices per revolution)

1992: Dual-slice spiral/helical CT
1 slice per revolution

1989: Single-slice spiral/helical CT
1 slice per revolution

Conventional CT

Hounsfield's CT Prototype

2 Major components of a CT scanner

Figure 2.1 Major system components of the CT scanner. These include the CT imaging system, the CT computer system, and the display, storage, and communication system.

Patient table

Gantry

Gantry aperture

Data acquisition → Image reconstruction → Image display, image storage, and image communication

X-ray imaging system

Computer system

Display, storage and communication system

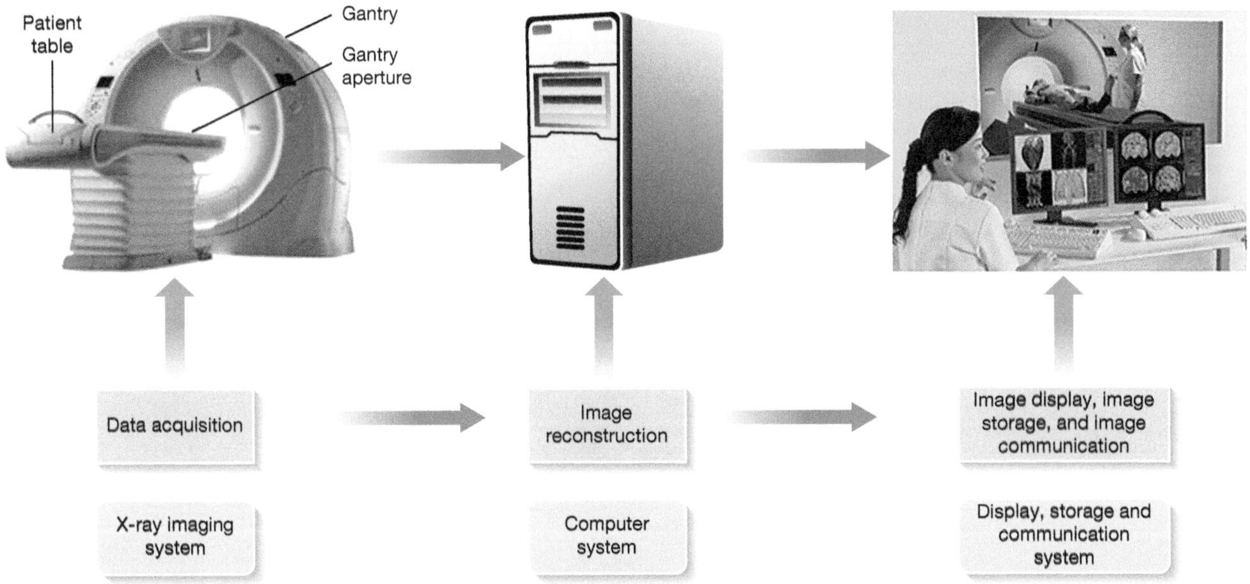

Figure 2.2 The essential components of a Picture Archiving and Communication System (PACS).

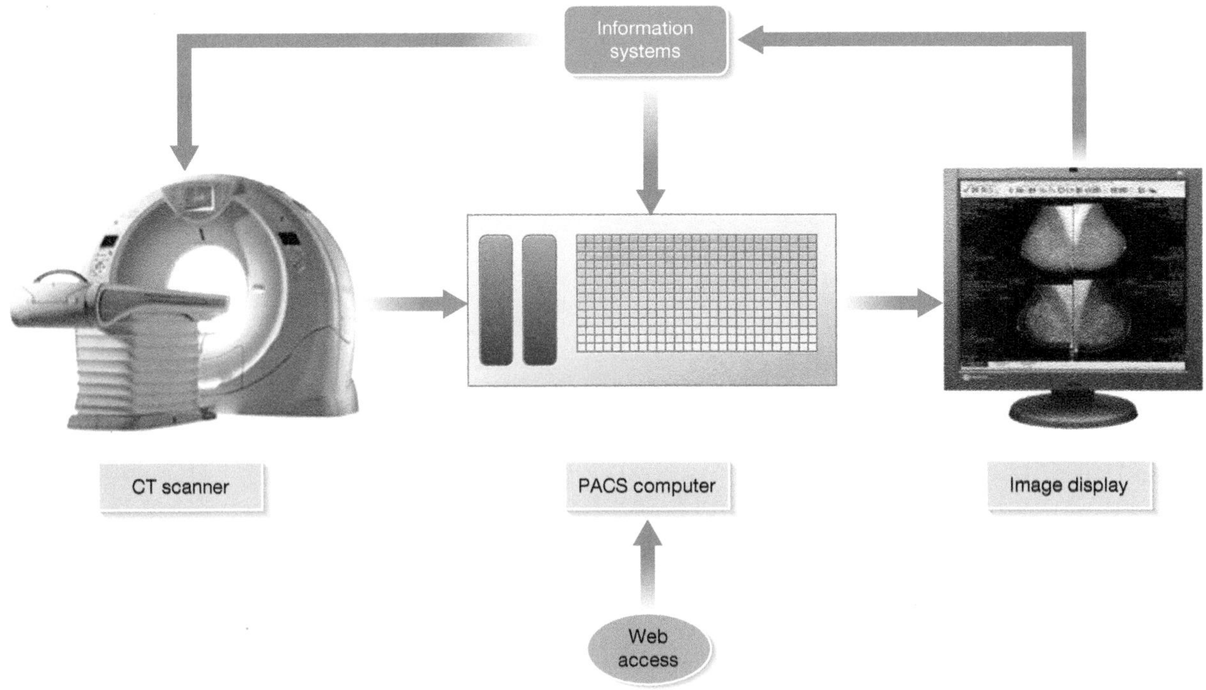

Information systems

CT scanner

PACS computer

Image display

Web access

CT at a Glance, First Edition. Euclid Seeram.
© 2018 John Wiley & Sons, Ltd. Published 2018 by John Wiley & Sons, Ltd.

Major system components

Figure 2.1, shows the major system components of a CT scanner. These include the CT imaging system, the CT computer system, and the display, storage, and communication system. Each system consists of specific equipment components that play a significant role in acquiring data from the patient, processing these data to create images, and subsequently displaying the images for viewing and interpretation by a human observer. Furthermore, these images can be recorded and stored for viewing at some later date, and can be sent to remote locations using computer communication networks.

The imaging system

The purpose of the imaging system is to produce x rays, shape and filter the X-ray beam to pass through only a defined cross-section of the patient, detect and measure the radiation passing through the cross-section, and convert the transmitted photons into digital information. This system consists of the X-ray generator, the X-ray tube coupled to detectors, and detector electronics, all housed in the CT gantry. The gantry itself includes an aperture, and the CT table, on which the patient is placed and positioned for scanning. During scanning the patient is moved through the gantry aperture as the X-ray tube and detectors rotate around the patient to collect X-ray attenuation data, or transmission readings. The X-ray attenuation data are converted to electrical signals by the detectors. These signals are then converted to digital data by the detector electronics. This process is called *data acquisition*.

The CT gantry must be capable of tilting to accommodate all patients and clinical examinations. The degree of tilt varies among systems, but ±12 to ±30 degrees in 0.5-degree increments is not uncommon.

The computer system

The computer is a central and integral component in CT, since it plays a major role in processing the data collected from the patient. Generally, computers are classified according to their processing capabilities, storage capacity, size, and cost. Currently computers are grouped in four main classes: supercomputers, mainframe computers, mid-range computers (minicomputers, an old term), and microcomputers. CT uses mid-range computers.

An important consideration is the *processing hardware*, which includes the central processing unit (CPU) and internal memory. The CPU is the brain of the computer; it consists of a control unit that directs the activities of the machine and an arithmetic-logic unit to perform mathematical calculations and data comparisons.

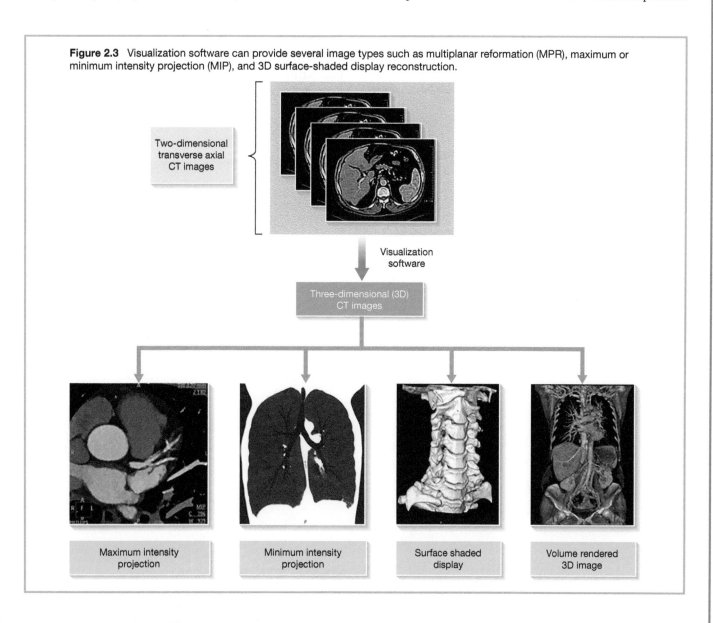

Figure 2.3 Visualization software can provide several image types such as multiplanar reformation (MPR), maximum or minimum intensity projection (MIP), and 3D surface-shaded display reconstruction.

In addition, the CPU includes an internal memory, or main memory, for the permanent storage of software instructions and data. CT scanners now use iterative reconstruction algorithms to reconstruct the image. These algorithms are complex and require increased computational power, which is now possible with the use of the *graphic processing unit* (GPU), and can be used to reduce the processing requirements of the CPU. The GPU is not within the scope of this book. CT image reconstruction is described in Chapter 10.

Display, storage, and communication system

The display, storage, recording, and communication are all part of what is referred to as the integrated console. This is a multimedia concept that allows the operator to have full control of the physical system, for example, gantry and table control. It also allows for real-time processing such as multiplanar reformatting, 3D manipulation, zoom, and pan. The integrated console controls the entire system and enables the operation of various functions. These are all part of the CT workstation (Figure 2.1), which features a display device with keyboard coupled to a microcomputer.

A display device for CT is generally a black-and-white or color monitor. These can be cathode ray tube (CRT) flat display or liquid crystal flat-panel display devices (Figure 2.1), with the latter now having generally replaced the former. The image is displayed in varying shades of gray and can be manipulated electronically to suit the viewing needs of the observer. CT examinations generate large amounts of data, hence large storage space in the order of gigabytes (GB) is required. Storage devices for CT include magnetic tape and disks, digital videotape, optical disks, and optical tape. Note that the capacity of an optical disk is much greater than that of magnetic tapes. Today, CD writers can be used for archiving CT images as well. Communications refer to electronic networking or connectivity by using a local-area or wide-area network (LAN or WAN). *Connectivity* ensures the transfer of data and images from multivendor and multimodality equipment according to a defined standard. A popular standard for medical images is the Digital Imaging and Communications (DICOM) standard. CT scanners are now connected to the Picture Archiving and Communications Systems (PACS). A basic PACS framework is shown in Figure 2.2 (to be described in more detail later).

CT software

In general there are three software categories for use in CT: reconstruction software, preprocessing software, and image postprocessing software. Reconstruction software are algorithms that build up the image from the raw data collected from the detectors; preprocessing software performs corrections (such as a bad detector reading) on the data collected from the detectors before the data are sent to the computer. Image postprocessing software operates on reconstructed images displayed for viewing and interpretation. Examples of such software include visualization and analysis software. Visualization software can provide several image types such as multiplanar reformation (MPR), maximum or minimum intensity projection (MIP), and 3D surface-shaded display reconstruction, as illustrated in Figure 2.3.

How CT scanners work

Figure 3.1 Essential steps in the production of a CT image.

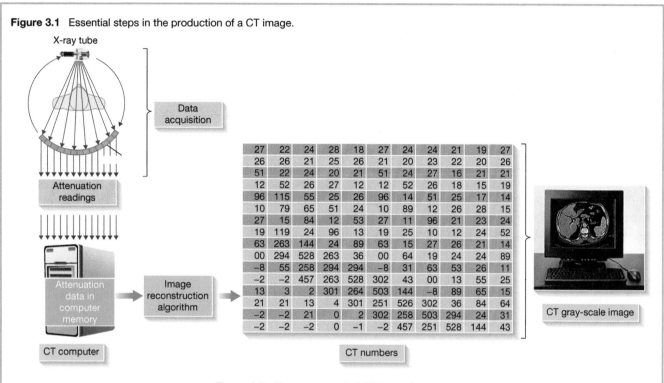

Figure 3.2 The reconstructed CT image is a numerical image. These numbers are referred to as *CT numbers*.

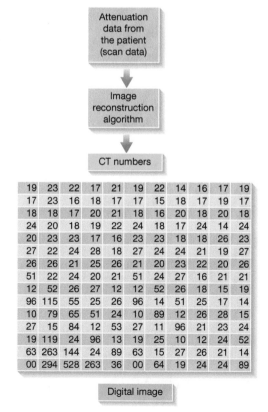

CT at a Glance, First Edition. Euclid Seeram.
© 2018 John Wiley & Sons, Ltd. Published 2018 by John Wiley & Sons, Ltd.

Essential steps in the production of CT images

The workings of a CT scanner are complex and involve not only X-ray production and radiation attenuation physics, but also detector and detector electronics, image reconstruction mathematics, and image display, manipulation, and communications. In brief, however, the production of an image in CT is illustrated in Figure 3.1.

The following are essential steps:

1 The technologist turns the scanner on and performs a quick test to ensure that the scanner is in good working order (not shown).

2 The patient is placed in the scanner aperture and positioned for the particular examination (not shown).

3 The technologist sets up the technical factors at the control console (not shown).

4 Patient instructions follow and scanning can now begin (not shown).

5 During data acquisition, X-rays pass through the patient, and are attenuated and subsequently measured by the detectors. The detectors convert the X-ray photons (attenuation data) into electrical signals, or analog signals, which in turn must be converted into digital (numerical) data for input into the computer.

6 The computer then performs the image reconstruction process using a reconstruction algorithm selected by the imaging department.

7 The reconstructed image is in numerical form. These numbers are referred to as *CT numbers* as shown in Figure 3.2. This is an important point, which will be described in more detail in Chapter 8.

8 These numbers are converted into gray-scale images and displayed on a television monitor for viewing and interpretation.

9 The images and related data are then sent to the PACS (not shown in Figure 3.1). Finally, the image can be stored on optical disks.

The flow of data in a CT scanner

In Figure 3.3, several components are shown. These include the data acquisition components and X-ray beam geometry, the detectors and detector electronics, the raw data preprocessor, the host computer with fast access memory, high-speed array

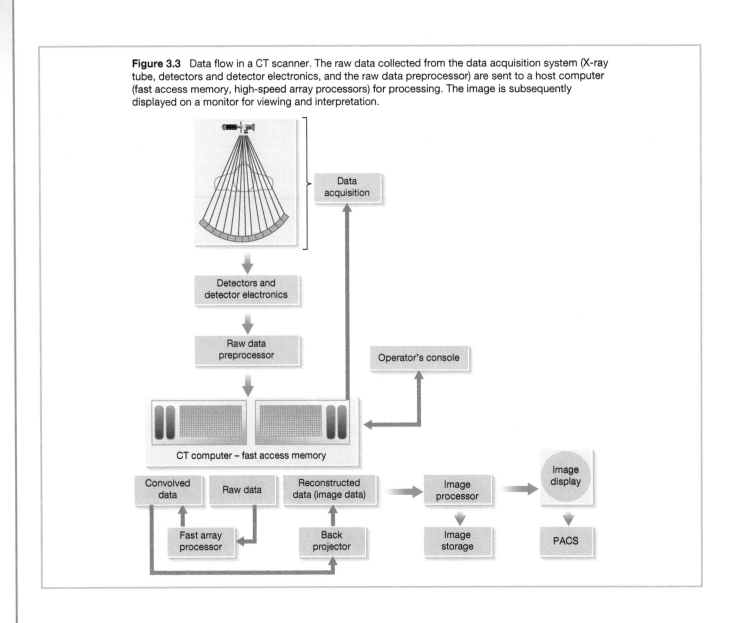

Figure 3.3 Data flow in a CT scanner. The raw data collected from the data acquisition system (X-ray tube, detectors and detector electronics, and the raw data preprocessor) are sent to a host computer (fast access memory, high-speed array processors) for processing. The image is subsequently displayed on a monitor for viewing and interpretation.

processors, digital image processor, storage, display, and operator's control console.

The flow of data from data acquisition to image display and communication, is as follows:

1 The X-ray tube and detectors rotate around the patient, who is positioned in the gantry aperture for the CT examination.

2 The radiation is attenuated as it passes through the patient. The transmitted photons are measured by two sets of detectors: a reference detector, which measures the intensity of radiation from the X-ray tube; and another set that records X-ray transmission through the patient.

3 The transmitted beam and reference beam are both converted into electrical current signals that are amplified by special circuits. This is followed by logarithmic amplification, in which the relative transmission readings are changed into attenuation (μ) and thickness (x) data.

4 Before the data are sent to the computer, they must be converted into digital form. This is done by the analog-to-digital converters, or *digitizers*.

5 Data processing begins. The digital data undergo some form of preprocessing, which includes corrections and reformatting.

6 The data are now referred to as *reformatted raw data*. Additional data corrections are performed by using computer software.

7 As shown in Figure 3.3, a special image processing operation known as *convolution* is performed on the data by the array processors.

8 The specific *reconstruction algorithm* then reconstructs an image of the internal anatomic structures under examination.

9 The *reconstructed image* can then be displayed or stored on magnetic or optical tape or disks. Finally, the images are sent to the PACS.

10 The control terminal is usually an operator's control console, which completely controls the CT system.

The technical evolution of CT

CT has experienced a number of significant technical innovations through the years, as illustrated in Figure 1.7. In brief CT has evolved from a scanner dedicated to imaging the brain in the transaxial plane only, to single-slice helical/spiral whole body scanners, and currently multislice helical/spiral scanners (all of which use one X-ray tube); and subsequently to scanners with two X-ray tubes coupled to two sets of detectors. The latter are known as dual source CT (DSCT) scanners. Other notable technical innovations include the development of multislice detectors, iterative reconstruction algorithms, virtual reality imaging methods, dose optimization methods, and important quality control test tools and procedures. These innovations are intended not only to improve image quality and reduce radiation dose, but also to play a role in the care and management of the patient, during CT imaging.

Advantages and shortcomings of CT

One of the most conspicuous advantages of CT compared with radiography, nuclear medicine, and ultrasonography is that CT offers the best low-contrast resolution (to be described later). For example, the contrast resolution (in millimeters at 0.5% difference) for CT is 4 compared to 10, 10, and 20 for radiography, ultrasonography, and nuclear medicine, respectively. Other advantages will be described in later chapters. A major disadvantage of CT is poor spatial resolution (detail measured in line pairs per millimeter) compared to other imaging modalities. For example, the spatial resolution for CT is 0.5, while for nuclear medicine, ultrasonography, and magnetic resonance imaging (MRI), the spatial resolution is 5, 2, and 0.5, respectively. Other disadvantages will be outlined in later chapters.

4 Data acquisition principles

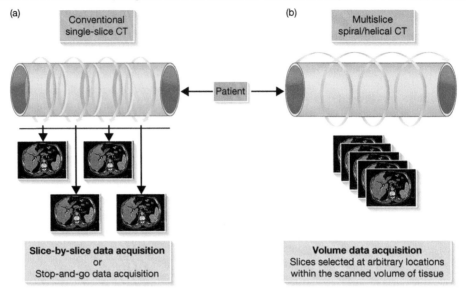

Figure 4.1 There are two methods of acquiring data from the patient: (a) conventional single-slice CT, and (b) multislice spiral/helical CT.

(a) **Conventional single-slice CT**

(b) **Multislice spiral/helical CT**

Patient

Slice-by-slice data acquisition
or
Stop-and-go data acquisition

Volume data acquisition
Slices selected at arbitrary locations within the scanned volume of tissue

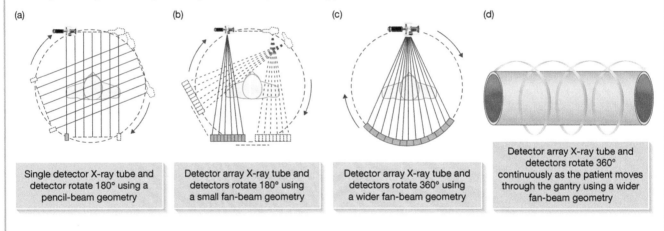

Figure 4.2 Three types of CT data acquisition beam geometries: the *pencil beam geometry* (a) and *fan-beam geometry* (b, c). The path traced by the X-ray tube during scanning describes a spiral or helix (d).

(a) Single detector X-ray tube and detector rotate 180° using a pencil-beam geometry

(b) Detector array X-ray tube and detectors rotate 180° using a small fan-beam geometry

(c) Detector array X-ray tube and detectors rotate 360° using a wider fan-beam geometry

(d) Detector array X-ray tube and detectors rotate 360° continuously as the patient moves through the gantry using a wider fan-beam geometry

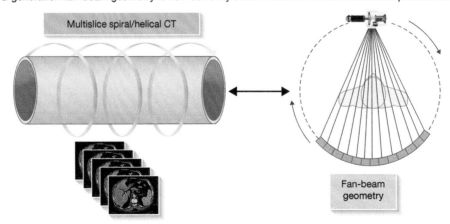

Figure 4.3 The third-generation fan-beam geometry is now currently used in state-of-the-art multislice spiral/helical CT (MSCT) scanners.

Multislice spiral/helical CT

Fan-beam geometry

CT at a Glance, First Edition. Euclid Seeram.
© 2018 John Wiley & Sons, Ltd. Published 2018 by John Wiley & Sons, Ltd.

Data acquisition methods

The final CT image is created from three technical and complex steps as illustrated in Figure 1.3. These include data acquisition, image reconstruction, and image display, storage, and communication. The first of these is data acquisition.

Data acquisition refers to the systematic collection of radiation attenuation measurements from the patient. These measurements (X-ray photons) are then converted into electronic signals, which are subsequently converted into digital data. These digital data go directly to the computer for processing, which results in the CT image.

There are two methods of acquiring data from the patient in CT scanning, as illustrated in Figure 4.1. These include:

1 conventional single-slice CT, and
2 multislice spiral/helical CT.

Conventional *single slice CT* (Figure 4.1a) involves a *slice-by-slice data acquisition* using different beam geometries (size, shape, and motion of the beam and its path) to scan the patient. Essentially, the X-ray tube rotates around the patient and collects data from the first slice. The tube stops, and the patient moves into position to scan the next slice (also referred to as a *stop-and-go data acquisition*). This process continues until all slices have been individually scanned.

Multislice spiral/helical CT (Figure 4.1b) is characterized by the use of a special beam geometry referred to as *spiral* or *helical geometry* to scan a volume of tissue rather than one slice at a time.

This is sometimes referred to as *volume data acquisition*. In spiral/helical CT, the X-ray tube and detectors rotate continuously as the patient moves through the gantry and trace a spiral/ helical path to scan a defined volume of tissue, during a single breath-hold. The continuous rotation of the X-ray tube and detectors is made possible with the use of slip rings (to be described later). This particular method generates a single slice per one revolution of the X-ray tube and is often referred to as a *single-slice spiral/helical CT* (SSCT). To improve the volume coverage speed performance of SSCT, *multislice spiral/helical CT* (MSCT) is now commonplace for faster imaging of patients. MSCT scanners generate multiple slices per one revolution of the X-ray tube. MSCT scanners have developed from 4, 8, 16, 32, 40, 64, and 320 slices per revolution of the X-ray tube. MSCT principles will be described in detail later.

Data acquisition geometries

As mentioned above, the term beam geometry refers to the size, shape, and motion of the X-ray beam and the path it traces as the patient moves through the gantry during scanning. There are three types of CT scanner acquisition beam geometries, which are schematically shown in Figure 4.2: *pencil beam geometry* (Figure 4.2a); *fan beam geometry* (Figures 4.2b and c), and CT scanning in *spiral or helical geometry* whereby the path traced by the X-ray tube during scanning describes a spiral or helix (Figure 4.2d).

Figure 4.4 The major components of the CT data acquisition system (DAS) include the X-ray tube, the X-ray beam filter, prepatient collimators, and the detectors and detector electronics (analog-to-digital converters).

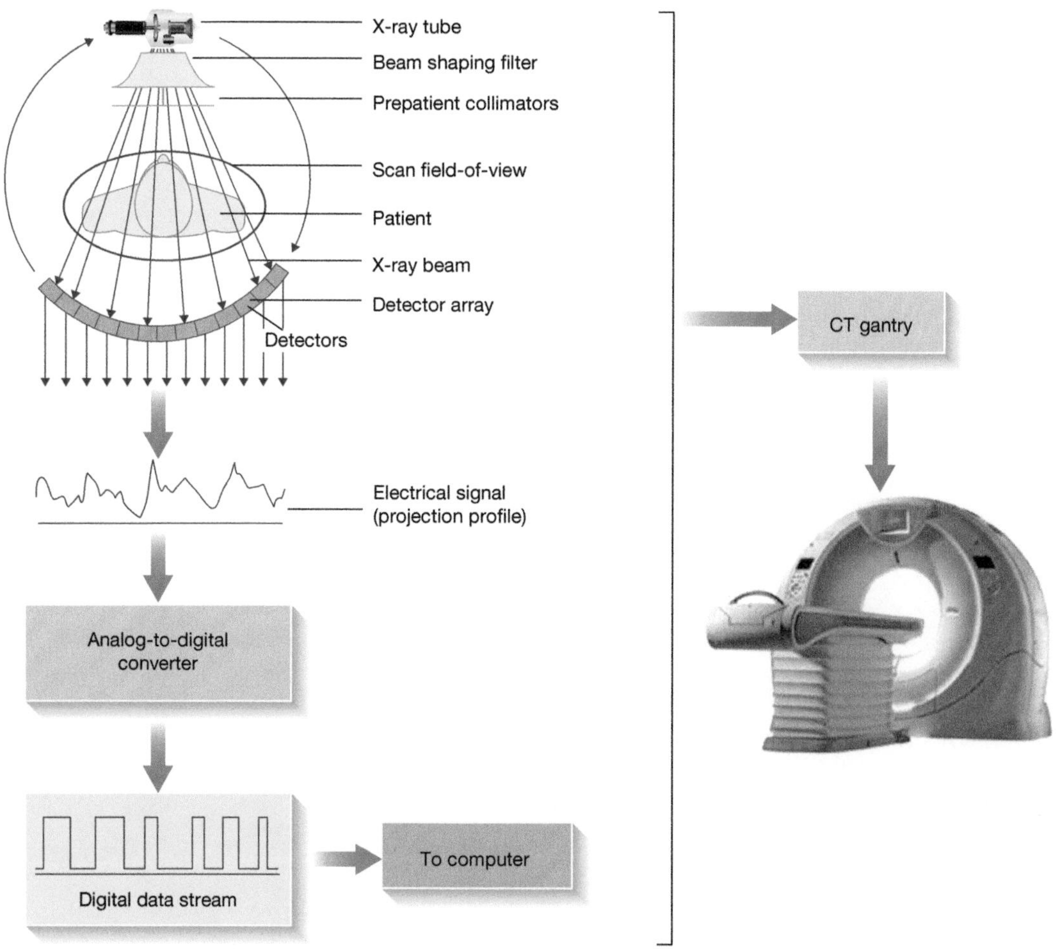

- X-ray tube
- Beam shaping filter
- Prepatient collimators
- Scan field-of-view
- Patient
- X-ray beam
- Detector array
- Detectors
- Electrical signal (projection profile)
- Analog-to-digital converter
- Digital data stream
- To computer
- CT gantry

The literature has identified seven generations of CT scanners. This categorization is based on the type of beam geometry used in the scanning of the patient. For example, first-generation geometry (Figure 4.2a) was used by Hounsfield and this was subsequently followed by the development and use of the second-generation (Figure 4.2b), third-generation (Figure 4.2c), fourth-generation, and so on. The third-generation fan-beam geometry is now currently used in state-of-the-art MSCT scanners (Figure 4.3). An important point to note is that the development of these different beam geometries provided the solution to faster scanning (shorter scan times) of the patient, and especially patients who are very sick and have the problem of holding a breath during the data acquisition. There is a mathematical relationship that states that the scan time is inversely proportional to the number of detectors. The more detectors used the shorter the scan time. Furthermore two MSCT scanners have been developed specifically for imaging the beating heart. These are the Toshiba Medical Systems Aquilion CT scanner family (320 slices per revolution of the X-ray tube and detectors) and the Dual Source CT (DSCT) scanner (Siemens Healthcare) designed for cardiac CT imaging because it provides the temporal resolution needed to image moving structures such as the heart.

Data acquisition components

The major *components* of the data acquisition system refer to those physical devices that shape and define the beam, measure its transmission through the patient, and convert this information into digital data for input into the computer as diagrammatically illustrated in Figure 4.4. These components include the X-ray tube, the X-ray beam filter, prepatient collimators, and the detectors and detector electronics (analog-to-digital converters). Each of these plays an important role in accurate imaging of the patient during CT scanning.

The following are essential steps in not only the arrangement of the components but also the process of acquiring the data from the patient:

1 The X-ray tube and detector are in perfect alignment.
2 The tube and detector scan the patient to collect a large number of transmission measurements.
3 The beam is shaped by a special filter as it leaves the tube.
4 The beam is collimated to pass through only the slice of interest.
5 The beam is attenuated by the patient and the transmitted photons are then measured by the detector.
6 The detector converts the X-ray photons into an electrical signal (analog data).
7 These signals are converted by the analog-to-digital converter (ADC) into digital data.
8 The digital data are sent to the computer for image reconstruction.

The components of the data acquisition are all housed in the CT gantry. More detailed descriptions will be provided in later chapters.

5 X-ray tubes and generator technologies

7

Figure 5.1 The X-ray generator provides high voltage to the X-ray tube for the production of X-rays. Generators used in a CT imaging system are high-frequency generators, which are very small and compact.

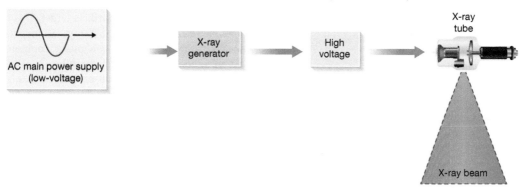

Figure 5.2 The essential electrical components of a high-frequency generator.

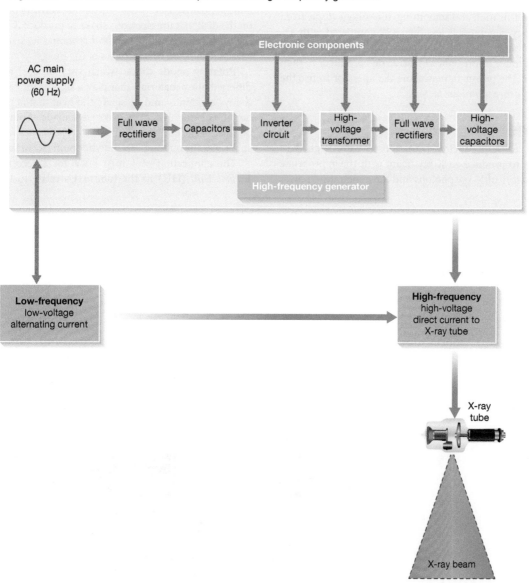

CT at a Glance, First Edition. Euclid Seeram.
© 2018 John Wiley & Sons, Ltd. Published 2018 by John Wiley & Sons, Ltd.

The X-ray generator

The X-ray generator is an integral part of the CT imaging system. The generator is coupled to the X-ray tube (Figure 5.1) via special electrical cables to provide high voltage to the X-ray tube. High voltage –as compared to the low-voltage alternating current (AC) from the main supply to the hospital or any other building – is necessary in order to produce X-rays. CT scanners now use very sophisticated *high-frequency generators*, which are small, compact, and very efficient in producing X-ray beams needed for imaging in CT. The high-frequency generator is now located inside the CT gantry and is mounted on the rotating frame with the X-ray tube. Both X-ray generator and X-ray tube rotate around the patient during CT scanning.

The components of a high-frequency generator are shown in Figure 5.2. It is beyond the scope of this text to describe the details of the high-frequency generator; however, the following points are necessary to understand how these generators work. First the *low-voltage, low-frequency current* (60 Hz) from the main power supply is converted to *high-voltage, high-frequency current* as it passes through the components. Secondly, each component changes the low-voltage, low-frequency AC waveform to supply the X-ray tube with high-voltage, high-frequency direct current of almost constant potential. The third point to note is that after high-voltage rectification and smoothing, the voltage ripple from a high-frequency generator is less than 1%, compared with 4% from a three-phase, 12-pulse generator. This makes the high-frequency generator more efficient at X-ray production than its predecessor. The power ratings allow the operator to use the appropriate *exposure technique factors*.

X-ray tubes

The exposure technique factors (mA and kV) are applied to the X-ray tube to produce an X-ray beam with the appropriate intensity – *quantity* of X-ray photons and the penetrating power (*quality*) of those photons. There are two types of X-ray tubes used in radiology: low-powered *stationary anode X-ray tubes* and the more high-powered *rotating anode X-ray tubes*. While the earlier CT scanners (first- and second-generation) used oil-cooled stationary-anode tubes, present day CT scanners use rotating-anode tubes.

The characteristic features of the rotating anode X-ray tube are illustrated in Figure 5.3. Also shown is a small part of the X-ray circuitry needed to control the mA and the kV applied to the tube and used for various examinations. X-rays are produced when high-speed electrons strike a target. This action results in about 98% heat and about 2% X-rays. To meet this requirement the X-ray tube consists of two major components, a cathode and an anode, both encased in a tube envelope that ensures a vacuum. The cathode assembly consists of mainly a thin tungsten wire wound in a helical fashion, called the *filament*, which is positioned in a focusing cup. When the filament is heated by a current (filament current) passing through it, it emits electrons by a process referred to as *thermionic emission*. The electrons are then accelerated to strike the anode. The flow of electrons across the tube is referred to as the *tube current* or *mA*. The acceleration of the electrons is brought about by establishing a *potential difference* (kV) between the cathode (negative electrode) and the anode (positive electrode). The anode consists of a target region on the disk that the electrons strike to produce X-rays. This small region is referred to as the *focal spot*, and its size influences the spatial resolution or sharpness of the image.

Rotating anode disks (which vary in size) are made up of different alloy materials that play a significant role in producing X-rays efficiently and dissipate the heat that is produced in the target. For example, early disks were made of pure tungsten, and because of the limitations in heat storage capacity, other materials such as rhenium tungsten molybdenum (RTM) are now used.

The application of 1 mA, 1 kV for 1 second will produce 1 *Heat Unit* (HU) in the tube. HUs relate to the *heat storage*

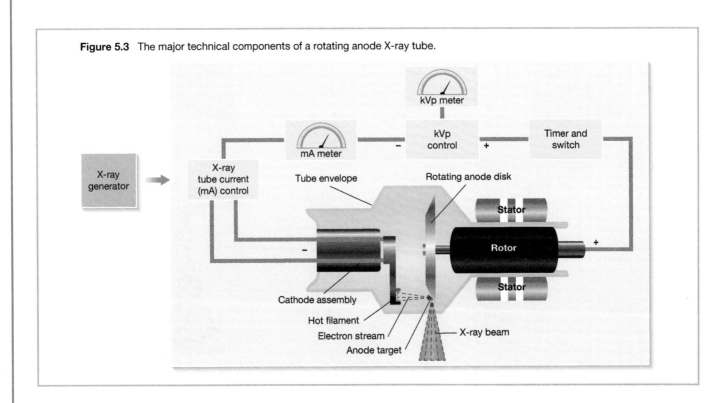

Figure 5.3 The major technical components of a rotating anode X-ray tube.

capacity of the tube. During operation of the X-ray tube, it is important to dissipate the heat produced so that the tube can be operated continuously and one does not have to wait for the tube to cool before another exposure can be applied. The tube envelope ensures a vacuum, provides structural support for the anode and cathode structures, and provides high-voltage insulation between the anode and cathode. Today tubes with metal envelopes are common, since they facilitate the use of larger anode disks and have higher heat storage capacities than their previous counterparts. For a more detailed description of the X-ray tube and its components, the interested reader should refer to the information provided at Perry Sprawls' online account of X-ray production (http://www.sprawls.org/ppmi2/XRAYPRO/#THE XRAY TUBE).

While the mA applied to the tube affects the quantity of X-ray photons produced, the kV affects the penetrating power (quality) of the photons. Furthermore, the dose to the patient is directly proportional to the mA and inversely proportional to the square of the kV. This will become important in Chapter 22 on dose in CT.

X-ray tubes for CT have evolved further to accommodate spiral/helical CT, which demands much higher X-ray output for longer scanning times. For example, the tube envelope, cathode assembly, anode assembly including anode rotation, and target design have all been redesigned. Such tubes are the Straton and the Vectron X-ray tubes (Siemens Healthcare) and the upgraded Maximus Rotalix Ceramic (iMRC) from Philips Healthcare (see manufacturers' websites for details).

6 X-ray beam filtration and collimation

Figure 6.1 A filter (e.g., a thin flat sheet of aluminum) is placed between the patient and X-ray tube to protect the patient by absorbing the low-energy X-rays that do not penetrate the patient (a). The CT filter (b) is a specially shaped filter (typically called a "bow-tie") designed to make the heterogeneous beam leaving the X-ray tube appear as a homogeneous beam at the detector.

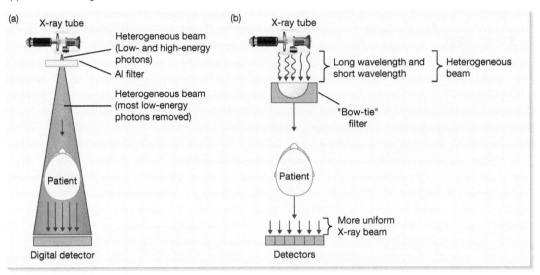

Figure 6.2 Filtration shapes the energy distribution across the radiation beam to produce uniform beam hardening when X-rays pass through the filter and the patient in a CT imaging system.

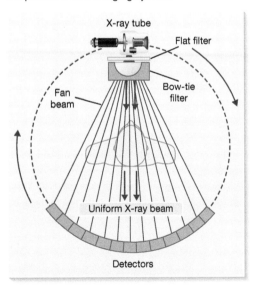

Figure 6.3 The basic collimation scheme used in CT. Adjustable *prepatient*, *postpatient*, and *predetector collimators* are necessary and important considerations in CT collimation.

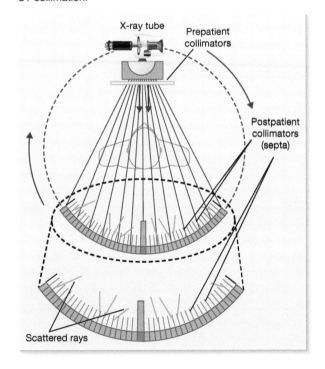

What is a filter?

The X-ray beam produced by an X-ray tube is *heterogeneous*, that is, the photons in the beam consist of both long and short wavelengths. While short-wavelength photons have high energy and hence more penetrating power, long-wavelength photons have low energy and less penetrating power. Consequently, high-energy photons penetrate the patient and reach the detector to create the image, whereas low-energy photons essentially are absorbed by the patient. Low-energy photons result in unnecessary dose to the patient.

Filtration in general radiographic imaging is intended to protect the patient from low-energy photons by removing them from the X-ray beam used to image the patient (Figure 6.1a). All X-ray tubes used in diagnostic X-ray imaging must have a certain amount of total filtration, which must comply with international and national radiation protection agencies, such as the International Commission on Radiological Protection (ICRP).

The CT filter

In CT, the filter is specially designed to ensure that the heterogeneous beam from the X-ray tube has the appearance of a *homogeneous beam* in order to satisfy the requirements of the CT image reconstruction process. This is illustrated in Figure 6.1b, which shows the heterogeneous beam (long and short wavelengths) from the X-ray tube being filtered by a *specially shaped filter* ("*bow-tie*") to provide a beam at the detector that is now more uniform (has the appearance of a homogeneous beam). It is important to note that Hounsfield used a homogeneous beam when he invented the CT scanner. This will become clear in Chapter 7, on radiation attenuation.

The purpose of filtration in CT is two-fold:

1 Filtration removes low-energy X-rays because they do not play a role in CT image formation; instead they contribute to patient dose. As a result of filtration, the mean energy of the beam increases and the beam becomes "harder," or more penetrating. This phenomenon, which is referred to as beam hardening, may result in beam-hardening artifacts.

2 Filtration shapes the energy distribution across the radiation beam to produce uniform beam hardening when X-rays pass through the filter and the patient, as shown in Figure 6.2. Furthermore, in CT the collimation is used to define the beam width for the examination.

X-ray beam collimation

In radiography and fluoroscopy, the X-ray beam is always *collimated* or *restricted* to cover only the anatomical area of interest. Such action results in reduction of unnecessary radiation to the patient. Therefore diagnostic medical imaging equipment must comply with the guidelines of the ICRP and related national radiation protection agencies.

In CT *collimation* is equally important because it affects patient dose and image quality. The basic collimation scheme in CT is shown in Figure 6.3, with adjustable *prepatient, postpatient,* and *predetector collimators*. An important consideration in CT collimation is that the detectors must be perfectly aligned to optimize the imaging process. Such alignment is accomplished with the fixed collimators, not shown in Figure 6.3. The collimators close to the X-ray tube and those close to the detectors are carefully positioned to ensure a constant beam at the detector. The collimators positioned close to the detectors also shape the beam and remove scattered radiation in an effort to improve image quality. The collimator section at the distal end of the collimator assembly also helps define the thickness of the slice to be imaged. Various slice thicknesses are available depending on the type of scanner. Some CT scanners employ an antiscatter grid to remove radiation scattered from the patient. This grid is placed just in front of the detectors and it is intended to improve image quality.

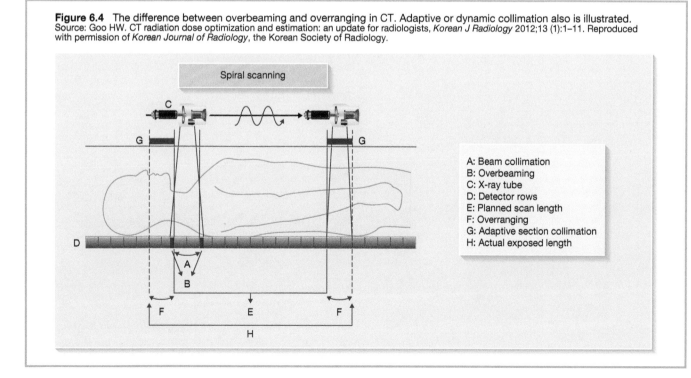

Figure 6.4   The difference between overbeaming and overranging in CT. Adaptive or dynamic collimation also is illustrated. Source: Goo HW. CT radiation dose optimization and estimation: an update for radiologists, *Korean J Radiology* 2012;13 (1):1–11. Reproduced with permission of *Korean Journal of Radiology*, the Korean Society of Radiology.

Spiral scanning

A: Beam collimation
B: Overbeaming
C: X-ray tube
D: Detector rows
E: Planned scan length
F: Overranging
G: Adaptive section collimation
H: Actual exposed length

Adaptive section collimation

The introduction of MSCT scanners posed some challenges with the design of the collimation scheme especially as the detectors become wider. The problems are related to what has been referred to as *overranging* and *overbeaming*, as illustrated in Figure 6.4. While overbeaming indicates that the beam is somewhat wider than the detector, overranging indicates that the patient is exposed to radiation beyond the needed length of the scan (at the beginning and end of the scan). As a result the dose to the patient is increased. Overranging, for example, can result in a 5–30% increase in the dose.

In order to address this significant problem, *adaptive section collimation* (Figure 6.4) was developed. By adjusting the collimators at the start and end of the scan, portions of the beam exposing the patient are blocked in the z-direction (z-axis, or longitudinal direction of the patient, as shown in Figure 6.4).

7 Essential physics: radiation attenuation

Figure 7.1 Radiation attenuation is the reduction of the intensity of a beam of radiation as it passes through an object (patient). The figure shows that of the photons entering the patient, 97% are absorbed or attenuated by the patient, and only about 3% are transmitted and reach the detector.

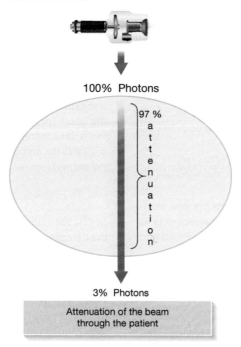

100% Photons

97 % attenuation

3% Photons

Attenuation of the beam through the patient

Figure 7.2 Attenuation of a homogeneous beam of radiation as it travels through water. See text for further explanation.

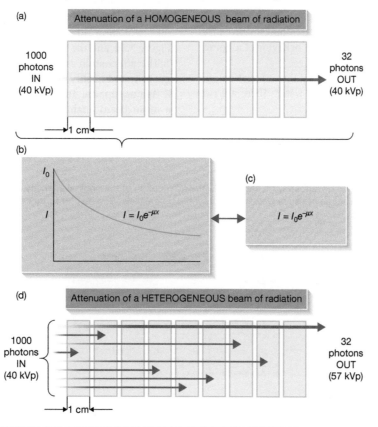

(a) Attenuation of a HOMOGENEOUS beam of radiation

1000 photons IN (40 kVp)

32 photons OUT (40 kVp)

1 cm

(b)

I_0

I

$I = I_0 e^{-\mu x}$

(c)

$I = I_0 e^{-\mu x}$

(d) Attenuation of a HETEROGENEOUS beam of radiation

1000 photons IN (40 kVp)

32 photons OUT (57 kVp)

1 cm

CT at a Glance, First Edition. Euclid Seeram.
© 2018 John Wiley & Sons, Ltd. Published 2018 by John Wiley & Sons, Ltd.

What is radiation attenuation?

The reduction of the intensity of a beam of radiation as it passes through an object is referred to as *radiation attenuation*, as illustrated in Figure 7.1. The figure shows that of the photons entering the patient, 97% are absorbed or attenuated by the patient, and only about 3% are transmitted and reach the detector. While some photons are absorbed, others are scattered. Radiation attenuation depends on the electrons per gram, atomic number, tissue density, and radiation energy used. Furthermore, there are two types of radiation beams (*homogeneous* and *heterogeneous*), and therefore a study of how each of these beams is attenuated is important to understanding the problem in CT. Attenuation in CT depends on the effective atomic density (atoms/volume), the atomic number (or proton number, Z) of the absorber, and the photon energy.

CT detectors measure the radiation transmitted through the patient from various locations. As a result, *relative transmission values* or *attenuation measurements* can be calculated as follows:

$$\text{Relative transmission} = \frac{\text{Intensity of x-rays at the source } (I_0)}{\text{Intensity of x-rays at the detector } (I)}$$

These attenuation values are sent to the computer and stored as raw data. A large number of transmission measurements are needed to reconstruct the CT image, and in general, several hundred views are required to reconstruct an image.

Attenuation of a homogeneous beam of radiation

In his original experiments, Hounsfield used a homogeneous beam of radiation. In a homogeneous beam, all the photons have the same energy, whereas in a heterogeneous beam (the X-ray beam produced by an X-ray tube, which is used in current CT scanners), the photons have different energies, and therefore it is important first to consider the attenuation behavior of a homogeneous beam.

Figure 7.2a shows what happens during the attenuation of a homogeneous beam as it travels through water. There are two important points to note about this:

1 Suppose that 1000 photons enter the block of water, and as a result of attenuation, 32 photons exit the water block. This is a reduction of the intensity of the beam (attenuation). In particular, the quantity of photons is reduced.
2 The initial beam energy (beam quality) has not changed. Photons enter the water block at 40 kilovolts (kV) and exit the block with the same 40 kV energy.

Not shown is yet another physical phenomenon with the attenuation of a homogeneous beam, and that is equal thicknesses of water sections (1 cm thick) remove equal amounts of photons. This is not the case with a heterogeneous beam.

The behavior of the attenuation of a homogeneous beam is shown in the graph, which shows exponential attenuation (Figure 7.2b), which can be described by the equation shown in Figure 7.2c. This equation is referred to as the *Lambert–Beer law*, where I is the transmitted intensity, I_0 is the original intensity, x is the thickness of the object, e is Euler's constant (2.718), and μ is the linear (per centimeter) attenuation coefficient. The objective in CT is to calculate the linear attenuation coefficient (μ), which indicates the amount of attenuation that has occurred. By taking the natural logarithm μ turns out to be:

$$\mu = (1/x) \bullet (I_0/I)$$

In CT, the values of I and I_0 are known (these are measured by the detectors).

Attenuation of a heterogeneous beam of radiation

The beam of radiation from an X-ray tube is heterogeneous beam and its attenuation through an object is very different to that of a homogeneous beam. In this respect, Hounsfield had to make several assumptions and adjustments to determine the linear attenuation coefficients.

Attenuation of a heterogeneous beam is illustrated in Figure 7.2d, and the following points are important:
1 The attenuation is not exponential, and as noted, both the quantity and quality of the photons change.
2 Again, suppose 1000 photons enter the block of water with a mean beam quality (energy) of 40 kV. Each block of water

Figure 7.3 The Lambert–Beer law describes what happens to the attenuation of the original intensity of photons (I_0) as a beam passes through tissues: (a) for a single volume of tissue (voxel) and (b) for multiple voxels. See text for further explanation.

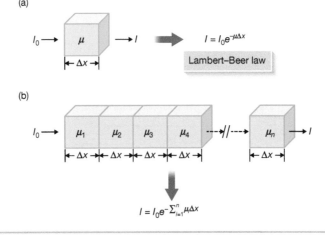

removes different quantities of photons, and the mean energy of the transmitted photons increases to 57 kV and 32 photons exit the block of water.

3 Lower energy photons are absorbed, which allows the higher energy photons to pass through. As a result, the penetrating power of the photons increases and the beam becomes harder.

Lambert–Beer law

The Lambert–Beer law is given for a single volume of tissue (voxel) as the input beam (I_0) is attenuated and the output beam, the transmitted beam (I) as illustrated in Figure 7.3a, is given by the equation:

$$I = I_0 e^{-\mu \Delta x}$$

For a length of tissue comprising of several voxels (Figure 7.3b) the attenuation is given by the equation:

$$I = I_0 e^{-\sum_{i=1}^{n} \mu_i \Delta x}$$

The equation $I = I_0 e^{-\mu \Delta x}$ applies only to a homogeneous beam. It then follows that in CT, which is based on the use of a heterogeneous beam, it is necessary to make the heterogeneous beam approximate a homogeneous beam to satisfy the equation. This was explained in Chapter 6.

8 Attenuation measurements and CT numbers

Figure 8.1 CT numbers are calculated from the attenuation readings or measurements stored in the computer after data collection. A CT number is an integer (0, positive number, or a negative number) and a CT image is made up of a number of integers, which represents a digital CT image.

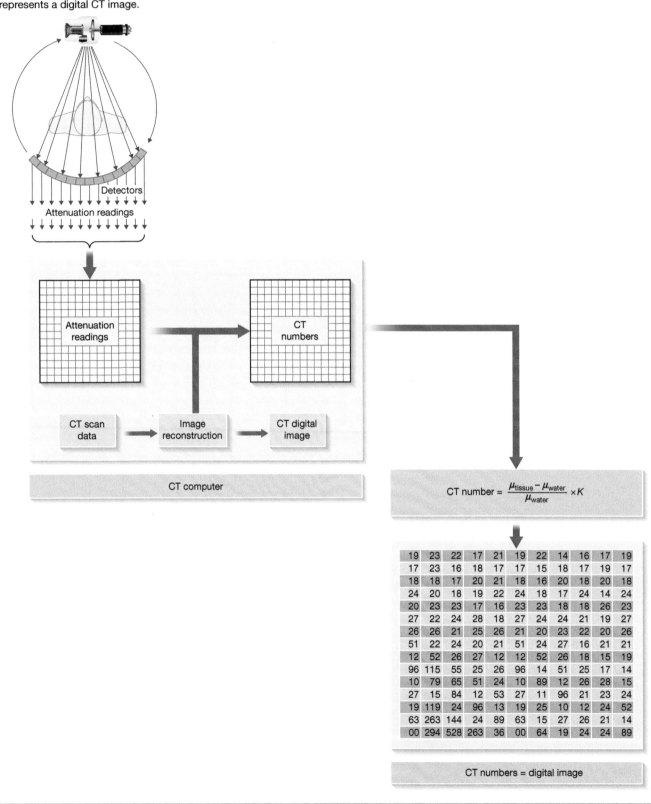

CT at a Glance, First Edition. Euclid Seeram.

© 2018 John Wiley & Sons, Ltd. Published 2018 by John Wiley & Sons, Ltd.

Attenuation measurements and CT numbers

The attenuation readings or measurements are stored in the computer and are used to calculate CT numbers as shown in Figure 8.1. A *CT number is an integer* (0, a positive number, or a negative number) and a CT image is made up of a number of integers, which represents a *digital CT image*. The CT image is reconstructed using a reconstruction algorithm.

The CT number is calculated from the attenuation measurements using the formula:

$$\text{CT number} = \frac{\mu_{\text{tissue}} - \mu_{\text{water}}}{\mu_{\text{water}}} \times K$$

where μ_{tissue} is the attenuation coefficient of the measured tissue, μ_{water} is the attenuation coefficient of water, and K is a constant. The value of K determines the *contrast factor*, or *scaling factor*. These numbers can be printed out and interpreted by an observer; however, radiologists and radiographers alike prefer a gray-scale image and thus the digital image must be converted into a *gray-scale image*.

An example of calculating a CT number is as follows:

1 Given the linear attenuation coefficients for bone and water to be 0.38 and 0.19 cm^{-1}, respectively, and the scaling factor (K) of the scanner is 1000.

2 Using the relationship shown above for calculating the CT number, the CT number for bone = 0.38 − 0.19/0.19 × 1000 = 0.19/0.19 × 1000 = 1000

The CT number for water would be 0.19 − 0.19/0.19 × 1000 = 0.

3 The CT number for bone is 1000, and the CT number for water is 0.

CT numbers and the CT gray-scale image

In Figure 8.2a, CT numbers are shown as a numerical image. This image must be converted into a gray-scale image (Figure 8.2d) because it is more useful to the radiologist than a numerical printout. This conversion requires that brightness levels – or *gray levels* (Figure 8.2b) as they are often referred to in digital image processing theory – be assigned to CT numbers. As seen in Figure 8.2c the upper (+1000) and lower (−1000) limits of the *gray scale* represent white and black, respectively. All other values represent various shades of gray. Furthermore, the gray scale can be manipulated by a technique called *windowing* to display shades of gray that the observer can actually see. Figure 8.2b shows 2000 numbers, with each representing a shade of gray. A human observer can only see about 40 shades of gray. Therefore it would be inefficient to display more than 40 shades of gray. Windowing allows the operator to display the image for effective viewing and interpretation. Windowing will be described in detail in Chapter 13. Finally the CT image is presented to the observer as a gray-scale image (Figure 8.2d).

CT numbers for various tissues

The gray level scale in Figure 8.2b is referred to as the Hounsfield scale, where bone is represented by a CT number such as +1000, air as −1000, and water as 0 CT numbers. The range of CT numbers for various tissues is shown in Figure 8.3. For example, while bone has a range of CT numbers from 800 to 3000; muscle has a range of CT numbers from 35 to 50. The CT numbers for water, fat, and air are 0, −100, and −1000 respectively.

Knowing these values often becomes commonplace as CT operators and radiologists become more and more experienced in scanning patients.

Figure 8.2 CT numbers are shown as a numerical image (a). This image must be converted into a gray-scale image (d) because it is more useful to the radiologist than a numerical printout. This conversion requires that brightness levels or gray levels (b, c) as they are often referred to (in digital image processing theory), be assigned to the CT numbers. See text for further explanation.

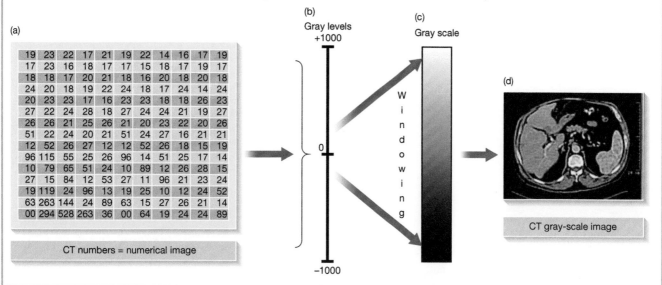

Figure 8.3 The gray level scale illustrated in (a) is referred to as the Hounsfield scale, where bone is represented by a CT number such as +1000, air as −1000, and water as 0 CT numbers. The range of CT numbers for various tissues is shown in (b).

(a)

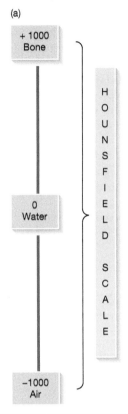

(b)

Tissues	CT numbers
Bone	800–3000
Blood (clotted)	55–75
Muscle	35–50
Brain (white matter)	36–46
Cerebellum	30
Brain (gray matter)	20–40
Blood	13–18
Cerebrospinal fluid	15
Tumors	5–35
Water	0
Fat	−100
Lungs	−150 to −400
Air	−1000

CT detector technology basics

Figure 9.1 The location of the CT detectors in the CT imaging system. As is clearly shown, the CT detectors are coupled to what is referred to as the detector electronics, which essentially consist of the analog- to-digital converters (ADCs).

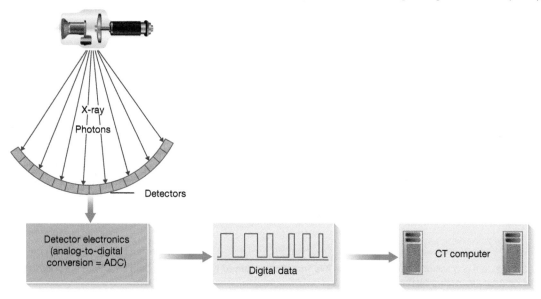

Figure 9.2 The major components of three types of detectors: (a) energy integrating detector, (b) dual layer detector, and (c) direct conversion detector, used in CT. See text for further explanation.

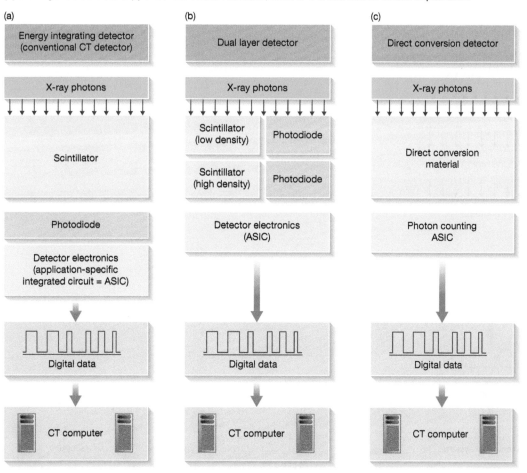

CT at a Glance, First Edition. Euclid Seeram.
© 2018 John Wiley & Sons, Ltd. Published 2018 by John Wiley & Sons, Ltd.

Location and purpose of the CT detectors

The *location* of the CT detectors in the CT imaging system is shown in Figure 9.1. As is clearly shown, the CT detectors are coupled to what is referred to as the detector electronics, which essentially consist of the analog-to-digital converters (ADCs).

The *purpose* of the CT detectors is two-fold; firstly, the detectors capture the transmitted X-rays from the patient, and secondly, these X-ray photons are converted into digital data by the ADCs. Subsequently the digital data are sent to the CT computer for processing such as image reconstruction using special algorithms.

Characteristics of CT detectors

In order for CT detectors to be effective and efficient in contributing to the production of good image quality, they must exhibit at least the following four characteristics. These include efficiency, stability, response time and dynamic range. While *efficiency* refers to the ability to capture, absorb, and convert X-ray photons to electrical signals, *stability* refers to the steadiness of the detector response. If the system is not stable, frequent calibrations are required to render the signals useful. Furthermore, *response time* of the detector refers to the speed with which the

detector can detect an X-ray event and recover to detect another event. Additionally, the *dynamic range* of a CT detector is the "ratio of the largest signal to be measured to the precision of the smallest signal to be discriminated (i.e., if the largest signal is 1 μA and the smallest signal is 1 nA, the dynamic range is 1 million to 1)" (Parker & Stanley, 1981). The dynamic range for most CT scanners is about 1 million to 1. Finally, *afterglow* refers to the persistence of the image even after the radiation has been turned off. CT detectors should have low afterglow values.

Types of detectors

There are three types of detectors used in CT: the *energy integration (EI) detector* (conventional CT detector, the more common of CT detectors), the *dual layer detector*, and the *direct conversion detector*. The latter will not be described any further in this chapter

The overall structure of each of these detectors is illustrated in Figure 9.2. It is clear that all three of these detectors convert X-ray photons to electrical energy and subsequently to digital data. Only the first two detector types (*scintillation detectors*) will be described briefly, since they are now commonplace in CT systems.

Figure 9.3 The data acquisition system, or DAS as it is sometimes referred to, converts analog data from the photodiodes into digital data for processing by the computer.

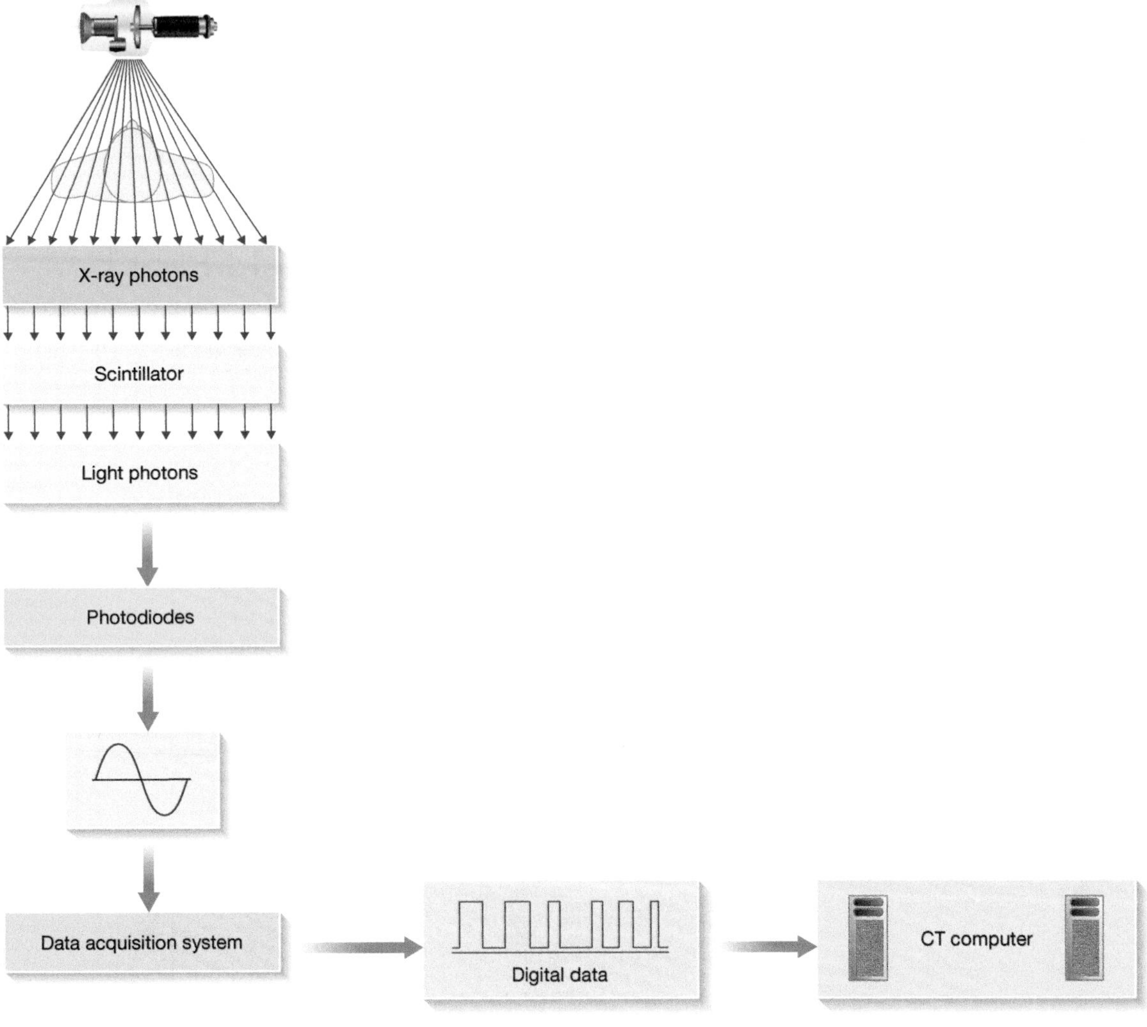

The EI detector features a scintillation crystal coupled to a photodiode (Figure 9.2a). While the crystal converts X-ray photons into light photons, the photodiode converts light into electrical signals. These signals are then digitized and sent to the CT computer for image reconstruction and image production. In the past sodium iodide, calcium fluoride, and bismuth germinate scintillation crystals were used. Today *cadmium tungstate* and a *ceramic material* made of high-purity, rare earth oxides based on doped rare earth compounds such as yttria and gadolinium oxysulfide ultrafast ceramic (UFC) are used. More recently lutetium (Lu)-based garnet has been introduced for use in CT. Generally these scintillators are used to improve the performance efficiency of the detectors in order to improve image quality in low-dose CT imaging, and reduce image artifacts.

The other detector type used in CT is the dual-layer detector (Figure 9.2b), made up of two layers of scintillators: a top layer of low-density scintillator (ZnSe), which absorbs low-energy X-ray photons that are subsequently converted to light photons; and a bottom layer of high-density scintillator (gadolinium oxysulfide), which absorbs high-energy X-ray photons that are subsequently converted to light photons. Both top and bottom scintillators are coupled to a vertically positioned thin front-illuminated photodiode (FIP), which converts light into electrical signals; the FIP is placed under the scattered radiation grid, so it will not compromise the detector's geometric efficiency. Furthermore, the dual-layer detector consists of an application-specific integrated circuit (ASIC) designed for the purpose of ADC, and integration of the two energies, that is, low- and high-energy spectra.

The materials used in the construction of this detector serve to ensure optimum performance in characteristics such as photon conversion efficiency, geometric efficiency, dynamic range, stability, linearity, uniformity, noise, and cross-talk, all of which influence the final CT image quality.

The data acquisition system

The data acquisition system, or DAS as it is sometimes referred to, is located as shown in Figure 9.3. The DAS is essentially the detector electronics, and its purpose is three-fold:

1 Measures transmitted radiation.
2 Encodes these measurements into binary data.
3 Transmits binary data to the digital computer.

10 CT image reconstruction basics

Figure 10.1 The attenuation data collected from scanning the patient at different angles is first converted to projection profiles.

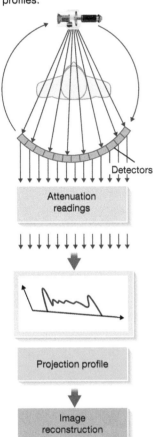

Figure 10.3 The back projection (BP) algorithm (a) produces a blurred image and therefore the filtered back projection (FBP) algorithm was introduced to solve this problem. A significant essential step of the FBP method includes the use of a one-dimensional (1D) digital filter called a convolution filter, applied to the projection data before backprojecting (2D or 3D) the data to produce an image free of blurring (b).

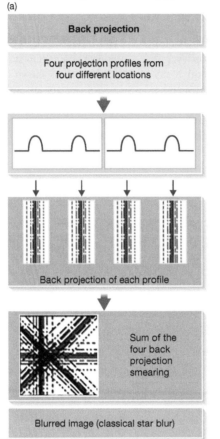

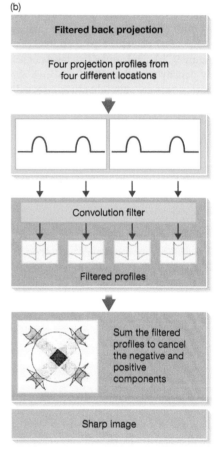

Figure 10.2 In the absence of an image reconstruction process (algorithm) the projection profiles produce an image that is referred to as a sinogram (not an image that can be used for diagnosis by radiologists) as shown in (a). With image reconstruction algorithms, the sinogram can be converted into a diagnostic image as shown in (b).

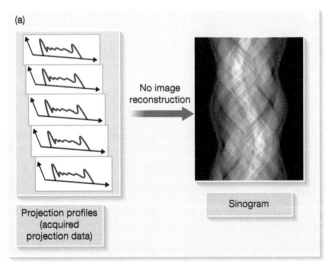

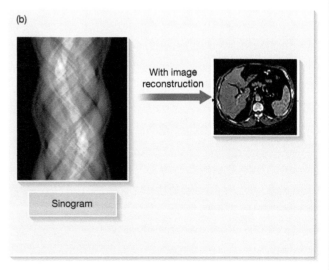

CT at a Glance, First Edition. Euclid Seeram.
© 2018 John Wiley & Sons, Ltd. Published 2018 by John Wiley & Sons, Ltd.

Major steps in CT

There are at least three major steps in the creation of a CT image, as illustrated in Figure 2.1. These include:

1 Data acquisition.
2 Image reconstruction.
3 Image display, image storage, and image communication.

The first of these steps, data acquisition, was described in Chapter 4. This chapter will address the second major step, image reconstruction. Chapters 11 and 12 will address fundamentals of image display, storage, and communication.

Image reconstruction basics

Definitions

This chapter will describe briefly only image reconstruction in *X-ray transmission CT* and not emission CT such as positron emission tomography (PET) and single photon emission tomography (SPECT).

Image reconstruction in CT involves complex mathematics to solve the fundamental problem in CT. This in itself is a mathematical problem, whereby the sum of the attenuation coefficients (line integrals) is solved by using an algorithm that performs the mathematics to calculate these coefficients (see Figure 7.3b). The attenuation data collected from scanning the patient at different angles are first converted to projection profiles as shown in Figure 10.1.

In the absence of an image reconstruction process (algorithm) the projection profiles produce an image that is referred to as a *sinogram* (not an image that can be used for diagnosis by radiologists), as shown in Figure 10.2a.

With image reconstruction algorithms, the sinogram can be converted into a diagnostic image, as shown in Figure 10.2b. An *algorithm* is defined as a finite set of very specific rules for solving a problem, such as the problem in CT.

Categories of reconstruction algorithms

In clinical practice, there are two categories of reconstruction algorithms, namely *analytical methods* and *iterative methods*. Analytical methods include Back Projection (BP) and Filtered Back Projection (FBP) algorithms. The most basic approach of the BP algorithm is illustrated in Figure 10.3a. This algorithm produces a blurred image and therefore the FBP algorithm was introduced to solve this problem. A significant essential step of the FBP method includes the use a one-dimensional (1D) digital filter, called a convolution filter, applied to the projection data before backprojecting (2D or 3D) the data to produce an image free of blurring, as illustrated in Figure 10.3b. The FBP algorithm became the workhorse of CT scanning until the late 1990s and early 2000s, when multislice CT (MSCT) scanners were introduced.

The BFP algorithms are not very accurate when used with the new generation of MSCT scanners, so other image reconstruction algorithms were introduced. These algorithms are called *cone-beam algorithms*. These algorithms are not within the scope of this text and therefore they will not be described here.

Iterative algorithms

It is well known that the FBP algorithm is not without its limitations, which include noise and streak artifacts. In particular, low-dose CT imaging – low mAs (milliampere seconds) techniques – produces noisy images. Typical artifacts with the FBP algorithm include metal artifacts and beam hardening artifacts, for example. These limitations require other approaches to reduce the noise, without compromising image quality (low contrast detectability and spatial resolution). There are several approaches available, such as the use of smoothing digital filters (with the FBP algorithm) and *iterative reconstruction (IR) algorithms*, for example.

Two major goals of IR algorithms are to reduce image noise (with the use of low exposure factors) and to minimize the radiation dose to patients. These IR algorithms have proved to be effective in that currently all CT vendors offer a variety of IR algorithms with their CT scanners. For example, while GE Healthcare offers Adaptive Statistical Iterative Reconstruction (ASIR) and Model-Based Iterative Reconstruction (MBIR), Siemens Healthineers offers Iterative Reconstruction in Image Space (IRIS) and Sinogram Affirmed Iterative Reconstruction (SAFIRE). On the other hand, Philips Healthcare and Toshiba America Medical Systems offer iDose and Adaptive Iterative Dose Reduction (AIDR), respectively.

The details of each of these are beyond the scope of this chapter; however, the basic idea of an IR algorithm is shown in a flowchart in Figure 10.4. The following steps are noteworthy in order to understand how an IR algorithm works:

1 *Measured projection data* are obtained and reconstructed using the FBP algorithm to generate the initial CT image (estimate). As can be seen this image is noisy.
2 This *initial image estimate* is then forward-projected to create *artificial raw data*, which is then compared with the measured projection data.
3 The *difference* between the two sets of data is calculated to generate an updated image (current CT image). The goal of the algorithm is to keep the difference between the current image and the measured projection data as small as possible. Such value requires the user to establish an *image quality criterion* to be used by the algorithm.
4 If the current CT image meets the required image quality criterion (IQC) then the process is completed and this image is now less noisy that the initial image.
5 If the IQC is not met, the *iteration process* is then repeated several times in what is known as the *IR loop*, until the difference is considered to be sufficiently minimal. The final CT image is a good quality image after the termination of the *iterative cycle*.

Note the visual comparison of the initial CT image generated with the FBP algorithm and the IR generated CT phantom image as shown in Figure 10.4. It is clear that the IR image has less noise than the initial CT image.

Figure 10.4 The major steps of an iterative reconstruction (IR) algorithm as outlined in the flowchart. See text for further explanation.

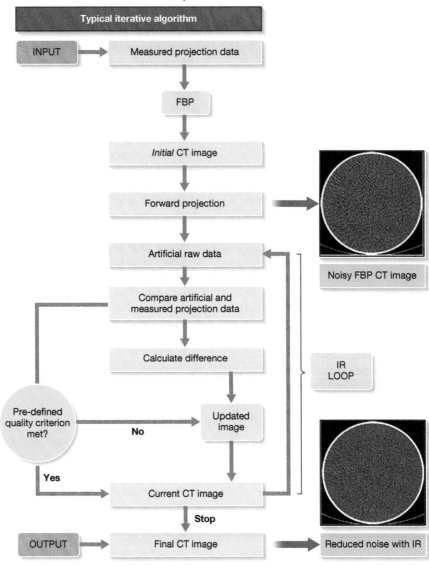

11 CT image display and storage

Figure 11.1 After the CT image has been reconstructed, it exits the computer in digital form (a). This numerical image must be converted into a form that is suitable for viewing and meaningful to the observer. Images in radiology are usually displayed as *gray-scale images* on a television monitor (cathode ray tube) (b) or liquid crystal display flat-panel devices (a).

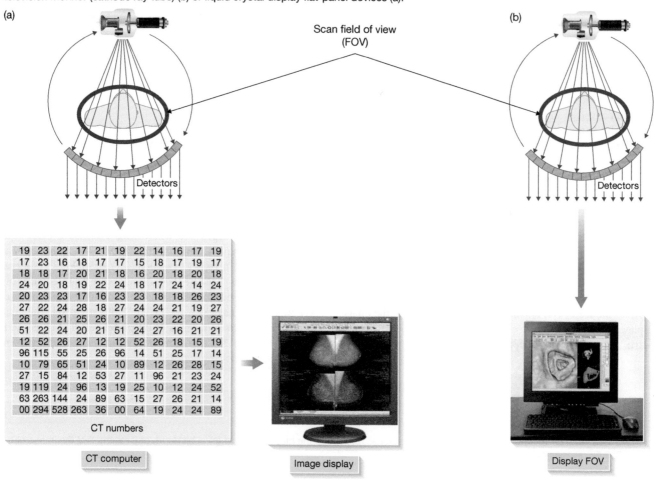

Figure 11.2 Spatial resolution in CT is related to the size of the pixel matrix, or matrix size.

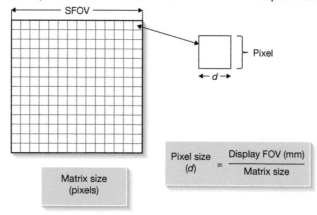

$$\text{Pixel size } (d) = \frac{\text{Display FOV (mm)}}{\text{Matrix size}}$$

CT at a Glance, First Edition. Euclid Seeram.
© 2018 John Wiley & Sons, Ltd. Published 2018 by John Wiley & Sons, Ltd.

Three major systems in ct imaging

The major systems in CT imaging are shown in Figure 3.1. The first system is the *data acquisition system*, which contains the X-ray tube, detectors, and detector electronics all housed in the CT gantry. This system collects attenuation data from the patient. The second component system is the *computer system*, which plays a major role in image reconstruction, image processing, and other applications. The third component is the *image display, storage, and picture archiving and communication system (PACS)*. The elements of this latter system are the basis for this chapter.

Image display characteristics

After the CT image has been reconstructed, it exits the computer in digital form, as shown in Figure 11.1a. This numerical image must be converted into a form that is suitable for viewing and meaningful to the observer. Images in radiology are usually displayed *as gray-scale images* on a television monitor (cathode ray tube as shown in Figure 11.1b) or liquid crystal display flat-panel devices (Figure 11.1a), with the latter replacing the former.

Although images are usually displayed in gray scale, non-image data such as text fields, patient data, and option selections can be displayed in color. Two noteworthy points here are the *scan field of view* (SFOV), or *reconstruction circle* as it is sometimes referred to, and the display *FOV* (DFOV). As shown in Figure 11.1a, the SFOV is the anatomical area being scanned by the CT scanner and it is subsequently displayed on the monitor as the DFOV (Figure 11.1b). The display FOV can be equal to or less than the scan FOV. Furthermore, other features of the image display system of importance in this chapter include the display matrix, pixel size, and bit depth.

Optimization of the displayed image fidelity (i.e., the faithfulness with which the device can display the image) is influenced by physical characteristics such as luminance, resolution, noise, and dynamic range. These topics are beyond the scope of this chapter. *Spatial resolution*, however, is an important physical parameter of the gray-scale display monitor and is related to the size of the pixel matrix, or *matrix size* (Figure 11.2). The *display matrix* can range from 64×64 to 1024×1024, but high-performance monitors can display an image with a 2048×2048 matrix. The spatial resolution determines the sharpness of the CT image. The smaller the pixels in the matrix, the sharper the image appears.

The *pixel size* can be computed from the FOV and the matrix size through the following relationship:

$$\text{Pixel size } (d) = \text{Field of view/Matrix size}$$

For example, if the reconstruction circle (FOV) is 30 cm and the matrix size is 1024×1024, then the pixel size can be determined as follows:

$$\text{Pixel size} = 30 \times 10\,\text{mm}/1024 = 0.29\,\text{mm} = 0.3\,\text{mm}$$

The final characteristics of the CT image to be described here are the bit depth and windowing. First, each pixel in the CT image can have a range of gray shades. The image can have 256 (2^8), 512 (2^9), 1024 (2^{10}), 2048 (2^{11}), or 4096 (2^{12}) different gray-scale values. Because these numbers are represented as bits, a CT image can be characterized by the number of *bits per pixel*. CT images can have 8, 9, 10, 11, or 12 bits per pixel. The image therefore consists of a series of bit planes referred to as the *bit depth* (Figure 11.3a). The numerical value of the pixel represents

Figure 11.3 The CT image consists of a series of bit planes referred to the bit depth (a). In (b), a bit depth of 8 means that the image can have 256 (8^2) shades of gray.

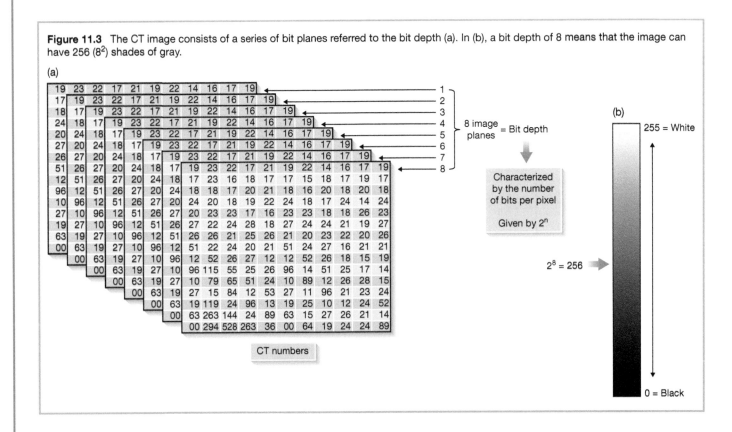

the brightness of the image at that pixel position. A 12 bits-per-pixel CT image would represent numbers ranging from −1000 to 3095 for a total of 4096 (2^{12}) different shades of gray. In Figure 11.3b, a gray-scale bar with 256 shades of gray is shown.

Windowing is an image processing operation whereby the CT image gray scale can be changed. Windowing is described in Chapter 13, on image postprocessing.

Image storage

CT images can be stored on magnetic tape and disks, digital videotape, optical disks, and optical tape. The choice of storage medium depends on several factors; however, optical disks can store much more data than magnetic tapes. A CT image of $512 \times 512 \times 2$ bytes (16 bits) would require 0.5 megabytes (MB) of storage. If the CT examination contains about 50 images, then 25 MB of storage is needed. If 50 examinations are performed in one day, then 1.25 gigabytes (GB) of storage is needed.

12 CT and picture archiving and communication systems (PACS)

Figure 12.1 Major system components of a typical picture archiving and communication system (PACS) configuration used in CT.

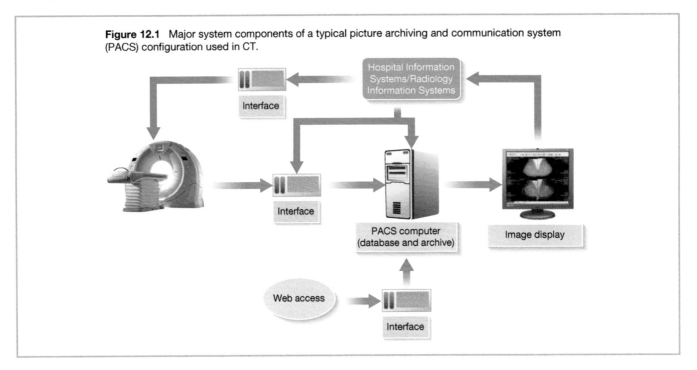

CT at a Glance, First Edition. Euclid Seeram.
© 2018 John Wiley & Sons, Ltd. Published 2018 by John Wiley & Sons, Ltd.

Electronic communications: basics

The number of images generated in a multislice CT examination can range from 40 to 3000, and the image size is $512 \times 512 \times 12$, hence one examination can generate upwards of 20 MB of data. Such vast amounts of data must be handled in such a manner that they can be easily displayed for viewing and interpretation, stored, and retrieved for retrospective analysis, Furthermore, they may be *transmitted* to remote locations within a healthcare facility, and to remote institutions, for the general management of the patient's medical condition.

After CT images are acquired by the operator they are sent to other systems such as storage or to a distant location. Radiologists subsequently access the examination images from storage to make a diagnosis. Sending these images to storage and other remote sites requires an *electronic computer networking* (connectivity) system using a local-area network (LAN) or wide-area network (WAN). *Connectivity* ensures the transfer of data and images from multivendor and multimodality equipment according to the *Digital Imaging and Communication (DICOM)* standard. The CT imaging system is therefore coupled to an electronic communication system, referred to as a picture archiving and communication system (PACS).

PACS: a definition

There are several definitions of PACS in the literature; however, they all identify certain technologies that characterize a PACS. For example, the main technologies include a computer system that integrates image acquisition, transmission, display, storage, data and report management, and information systems such as the *Hospital Information System (HIS)* and *the Radiology Information System (RIS)*.

Major components of a PACS

Figure 12.1 illustrates a typical PACS configuration for CT imaging, and consists of several major components. These technical components include the CT scanner coupled to what is often referred to as the *PACS controller*, via an electronic interface. This component includes a *database* and *servers*, such as the *image and archive servers* as well as *archival storage*. In addition, systems such as the RIS and HIS, image display, and a web server are all connected by various computer networks.

The first component of the PACS includes the image acquisition system, the CT scanner. Once the images are obtained by the scanner, they are sent to the PACS computer, which is a "high-end" computer or server, also referred to as the PACS controller, where they are stored and archived for retrospective analysis. The images are also displayed for subsequent interpretation. This computer workstation consists of hardware and software to facilitate the display of digital images for diagnostic interpretation and for review purposes. The PACS workstation is often referred to as a *soft-copy display workstation*.

Another important component of a large-scale PACS is a web server in PACS and it allows users to access images remotely, using *Internet browser technology* and microcomputers, which would allow access from within an institution or from outside the institution.

The functionality and usefulness can be extended by integrating the PACS with the RIS-HIS using computer networks. The devices within the PACS communicate with each other. Such integration and communication requires two *communication protocol standards*, which are essential to connectivity. While a protocol dictates exactly how certain tasks will be accomplished, a standard is a model and protocol that defines how products and services will be developed.

Communication protocol standards in digital radiology

The integration of the CT PACS with the RIS and HIS is based on two communication protocol standards, *health level 7 (HL-7) and DICOM*. HL-7 is the standard application protocol that deals mainly with text data, such as patient demographics, medical problems, and so forth, for use in most HIS and RIS systems; DICOM is the imaging communication protocol for PACS, and it deals mainly with image data, as well as limited amounts of text data. These protocol standards will not be described further in this book.

13 CT image postprocessing

Figure 13.1 The numerical CT image (a) is made up of a range of CT numbers called gray levels (b). These numbers are subsequently converted into gray scale (c). Windowing is a digital image processing technique in which the gray scale can be manipulated such that the operator (or observer) can alter these numbers to optimize the demonstration of the different structures, as shown in (d).

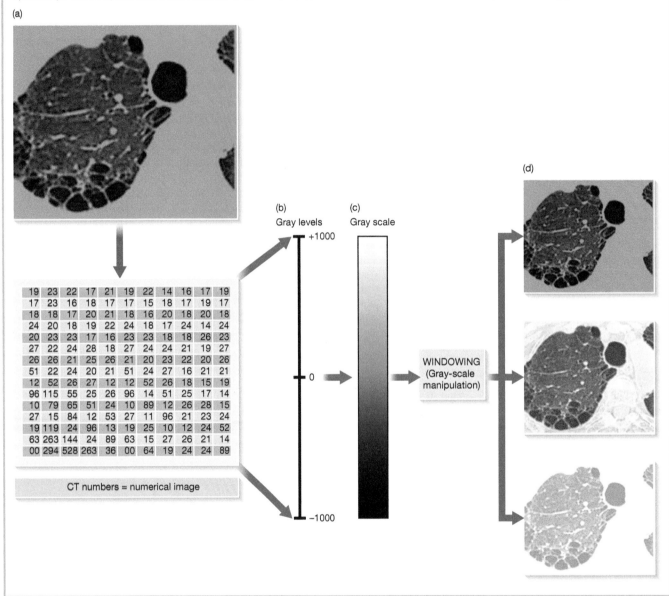

CT at a Glance, First Edition. Euclid Seeram.
© 2018 John Wiley & Sons, Ltd. Published 2018 by John Wiley & Sons, Ltd.

What is image postprocessing?

Image postprocessing has become an essential and common-place tool in digital radiology departments including CT imaging. *Image postprocessing* belongs to the domain of digital image processing whereby a number of digital processing techniques are used to modify the initial CT reconstructed images displayed for viewing and interpretation. These operations or techniques are used to change the overall appearance of the displayed image to enhance the visualization of structures in the image. For example, image characteristics such as brightness and contrast can be changed to suit the viewing needs of the observer. There are two categories of image processing, *linear* and *non-linear techniques*. While the former deal with image smoothing and image enhancement, the latter techniques are concerned with gray-scale manipulation, which modifies the gray scale of the image. This chapter specifically addresses gray-scale manipulation, commonly referred to as *windowing*.

Windowing overview

The technique of windowing is the most common image post-processing operation used routinely in CT. Windowing is also referred to as *gray-level mapping*, which is also popularly referred to as "contrast enhancement," "contrast stretching," "histogram modification," and "histogram stretching." The CT image is stored in the computer as a numerical image (Figure 13.1a), which is made up of a range of CT numbers called gray levels (Figure 13.1b). These numbers are subsequently converted into gray scale, with the lower numbers assigned black and the higher numbers assigned white (Figure 13.1c). In windowing, the CT image gray scale can be manipulated with the CT numbers of the image. The operator (or observer) can alter these numbers to optimize the demonstration of the different structures, as shown in Figure 13.1d. By manipulating CT numbers of various tissues, the picture can be changed to show soft tissues and dense structures such as bone. The picture contrast and brightness are easily changed with two control mechanisms: the window width (WW) and the window level (WL), respectively.

WW (Window Width) and WL (Window Level): definitions

The *WW* is defined as the range of the CT numbers in the image; it determines the maximum shades of gray that the displayed image can have. On the other hand, the *WL* is defined as the center of the range of CT numbers. Both of these are illustrated in Figure 13.2a, which shows a WW of 2000 (1000 + 1000) and a WL of 0. Furthermore, while Figure 13.2b shows a representation of the CT numbers for various tissues, Figure 13.2c illustrates the gray-scale display of the image ranging from black (lower CT numbers) to white (higher CT numbers). In addition, Table 13.1 lists typical WW and WL values used for

Table 13.1 Typical WW and WL values for different tissues.

Tissues	Window Width	Window Level
Temporal bone	3000	500
Spine	1600	300
Soft tissue (orbits)	400	30
Soft tissue (chest)	400	40
Abdomen	400	50
Brain (posterior fossa)	100	40
Soft tissue (cervical and thoracic spines)	500	60
Brain	80	40
Lung	1500	−400

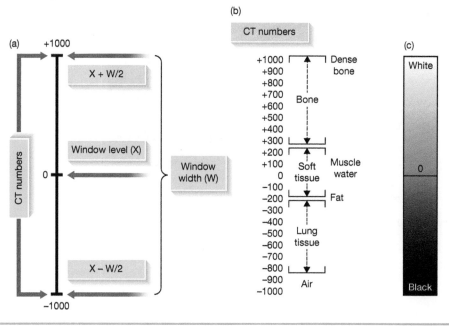

Figure 13.2 The definition of window width (WW) and window level (WL), as shown in (a). While (b) shows a representation of the CT numbers for various tissues, (c) illustrates the gray-scale display of the image ranging from black (lower CT numbers) to white (higher CT numbers).

Figure 13.3 The effect of three WW settings on image contrast (fixed WL): wide WW (a), medium WW (b), and narrow WW (c).

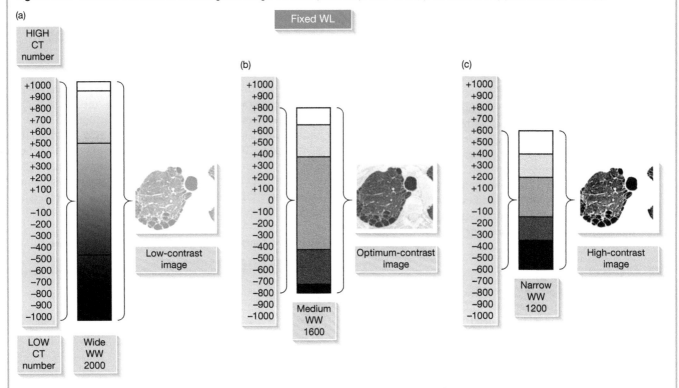

Figure 13.4 The effect of three WL settings on image brightness (fixed WW): high WL (a), medium WL (b), and low WW (c).

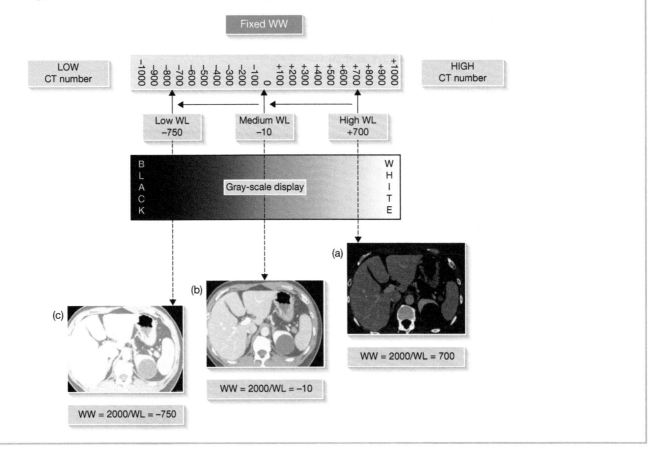

various tissues. Although Figure 13.2 shows a WW range of 2000 CT numbers, this range varies among CT vendors. While some scanners use a range from −1000 to +3095 (WW = 4095), other scanners use a range of −2048 to +6143 HU (WW = 8191).

Effect of WW and WL on visual image quality

The WW (contrast control) and the WL (brightness control) can be changed by the observer to optimize the image contrast and brightness. In Figure 13.3, while a wide WW (Figure 13.3a) produces a long gray scale (low-contrast image), a narrow WW (Figure 13.3c) results in a high-contrast image (short gray scale). Optimum image contrast is determined by the selection of the appropriate medium WW setting (Figure 13.3b); Table 13.1 guides this selection.

Figure 13.4 shows the effect of the WL on image brightness. Keeping the WW fixed (2000) as the WL increases (WL = +700) the image becomes darker, since more of the lower CT numbers (assigned black) are displayed. Furthermore, as the WL

decreases (WL = −750), the image becomes brighter, since more of the higher CT numbers (assigned white) are displayed. Again, Table 13.1 provides some degree of guidance in selection of the appropriate WL settings for the tissues being imaged.

Volume visualization image processing

With the advent of multislice CT (described in Chapter 14) leading to the collection of vast amounts of data from the patient during an examination, more and more sophisticated image processing methods have become available. These image data sets in the computer (*three-dimensional space*) are processed to generate three-dimensional (3D) images such as projection images (*maximum* and *minimum intensity images*), *multiplanar reformatted images, surface shaded images, volume rendered images,* and *virtual reality images.* CT vendors now offer basic and advanced 3D volume visualization software. These processing operations are beyond the scope of this book, and includes basic as well as advanced techniques.

14 Multislice CT – essential principles: part 1

Figure 14.1 In MSCT the path traced by the X-ray beam coupled with patient translation describes a beam geometry referred to as a spiral/helical geometry.

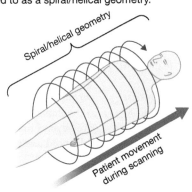

Spiral/helical geometry

Patient movement during scanning

Figure 14.2 While one-dimensional (1D) detectors are used in SSCT scanners (a), two-dimensional (2D) detectors are used in MSCT scanners (b).

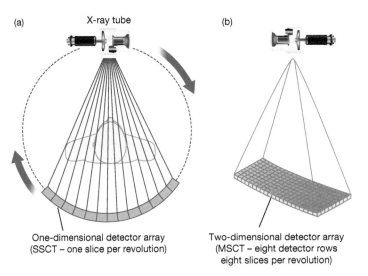

(a) X-ray tube

(b)

One-dimensional detector array
(SSCT – one slice per revolution)

Two-dimensional detector array
(MSCT – eight detector rows
eight slices per revolution)

Figure 14.3 2D detector arrays have been placed into two categories, the matrix array detector (a) and the adaptive array detector (b), the design of which is based on the vendor's preference.

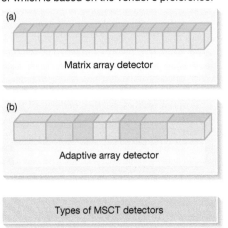

(a)

Matrix array detector

(b)

Adaptive array detector

Types of MSCT detectors

CT at a Glance, First Edition. Euclid Seeram.
© 2018 John Wiley & Sons, Ltd. Published 2018 by John Wiley & Sons, Ltd.

The essential principles of multislice CT (MSCT) include terminology, the technical requirements for MSCT, slip-ring technology, data acquisition, detector technology, image reconstruction, pitch, and selectable parameters. These principles will be described in two parts. Part 1 will focus on the evolution of scanners from the first scanner invented by Hounsfield, terminology, technical requirements for MSCT, slip-ring technology, and finally the advantages of MSCT compared to conventional CT (CCT) and single-slice CT (SSCT).

Evolution

Figure 1.7 is a flow diagram showing the evolution of CT, beginning with the first CT scanner designed by Hounsfield, which subsequently led to the development of other types of CT scanner designs. The evolution of the first prototype scanner, intended for scanning only the head, includes what has been popularly referred to as *CCT*, *SSCT*, and *MSCT*, leading to future scanner developments. While SSCT scanners acquire volume data sets and provide shorter scan times and improvements in 3D imaging compared to CCT scanners using a 1D detector array, MSCT scanners acquire volume data sets and have a volume coverage speed much faster than SSCT scanners using 2D detector arrays. It is important to note that some authors prefer to use the term multi-detector CT (MDCT). In this book MSCT terminology will be used.

Terminology

Increasing the volume coverage speed compared to "stop and go" CCT, the X-ray tube must rotate continuously around the patient while the patient moves through the gantry aperture during the scanning to cover an entire volume of tissue. The first concern is what happens to the image as the patient is moved through the

gantry aperture while the X-ray beam is on? The second point to note is that the path traced by the X-ray beam coupled with patient translation describes a beam geometry referred to as a *spiral/helical geometry* (Figure 14.1). While some vendors use the term "spiral" (e.g., Siemens Healthineers), others use the term "helical" (e.g., Toshiba Medical Systems).

CCT scanners use a *one-dimensional (1D) detector array* to scan one slice per rotation of the X-ray tube and detectors. SSCT scanners use a *1D detector array* (Figure 14.2a) and during data acquisition, only one slice is acquired per single rotation of the X-ray tube. To scan a volume of tissue (*volume scanning*), several rotations are needed, after which several slices and associated images are computer generated for the volume scanned during a single breath-hold. MSCT scanners, on the other hand, use a *2D detector array* (Figure 14.2b) to collect several slices per rotation of the X-ray tube. These 2D detector arrays have been placed into two categories, the *matrix array detector* (Figure 14.3a) and the *adaptive array detector* (Figure 14.3b), the design of which is based on the vendor's preference. While the former is divided into equal detector elements (14), the latter consists of pairs of elements that are equal (the central two elements are equal, the two closest to the central ones are equal, and so on). How each of these two types of detectors is used during data acquisition will be described in Chapter 15, which will focus on data acquisition for both SSCT and MSCT scanners.

Technical requirements for volume scanning

To acquire images with volume scanning, the following technical requirements are needed:

1 Continuous rotation of the X-ray tube made possible with slip-ring technology.
2 Continuous motion of the table during data acquisition.

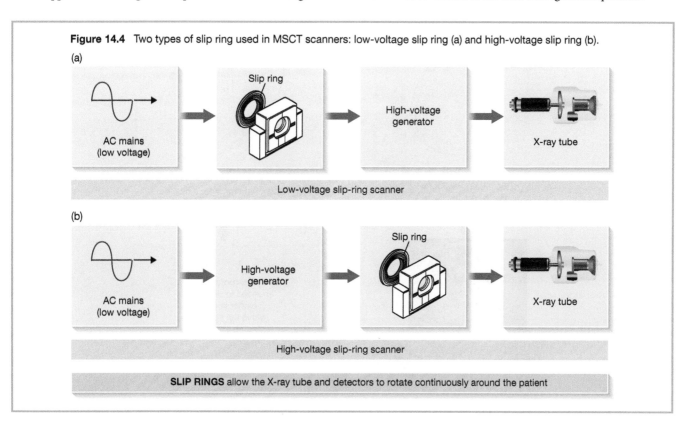

Figure 14.4 Two types of slip ring used in MSCT scanners: low-voltage slip ring (a) and high-voltage slip ring (b).

(a)

AC mains (low voltage) → Slip ring → High-voltage generator → X-ray tube

Low-voltage slip-ring scanner

(b)

AC mains (low voltage) → High-voltage generator → Slip ring → X-ray tube

High-voltage slip-ring scanner

SLIP RINGS allow the X-ray tube and detectors to rotate continuously around the patient

Figure 14.5 A comparison between slice-by-slice (a) data acquisition and spiral/helical volume (b) data acquisition. See text for further explanation.

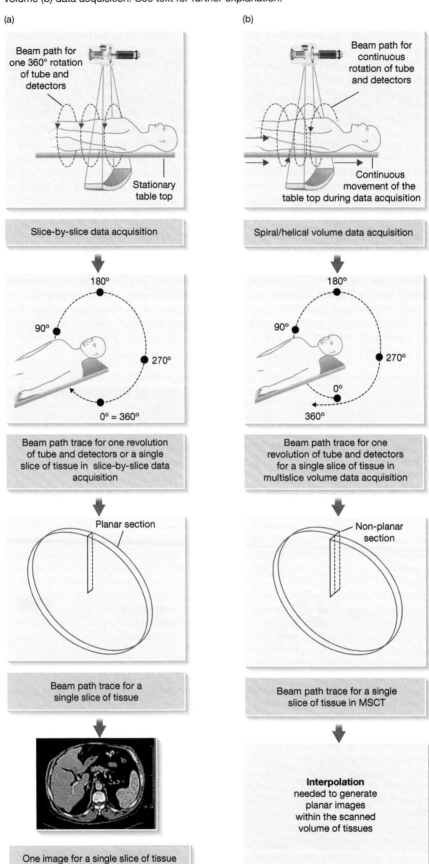

3 Increased electrical loadability of the X-ray tube (at least 200 mA per revolution is needed continuously throughout the time it takes to scan the volume of tissue).

4 Higher cooling capacity of the tube.

5 Special spiral/helical weighting algorithm.

6 Mass memory buffer to store the vast amount of data collected.

Advantages for spiral/helical technology

MSCT technology offers several advantages over CCT and SSCT. These include increased volume coverage speed, improved spatial resolution over SSCT, efficient use of the X-ray beam, reduced radiation dose to the patient, improved accuracy in needle positioning during CT fluoroscopy, and cardiac imaging.

Slip-ring technology

Slip rings enable the continuous rotation of the X-ray tube and detectors during volume data acquisition, by providing electrical power to the X-ray tube. Two types of slip-ring schemes are illustrated in Figure 14.4. These rings are electromechanical devices consisting of circular electrical conductive rings and brushes that transmit electrical energy across a rotating interface. While some vendors use a low-voltage slip ring (Figure 14.4a), others use a high-voltage slip ring (Figure 14.4b). In the latter approach, the high-voltage generator does not rotate with the X-ray tube.

Slice geometry during SSCT data acquisition

The essential steps to acquiring slices using a SSCT scanner are shown in Figure 14.5a, which shows the beam path for one 360° rotation of tube and detectors with the patient stationary. It is clear that a single slice of tissue is imaged using this beam geometry. The *planar section* is reconstructed (using the Filtered Back Projection algorithm) and displayed for viewing. SSCT scanners increase the volume coverage speed compared to CCT slice-by-slice scanners, but are now obsolete and have been replaced by MSCT scanners.

Slice geometry during MSCT data acquisition

The acquisition of spiral/helical CT scanners is illustrated in Figure 14.5b. The tube and detectors rotate around the patient, who is moving at the same time in order to scan a volume of tissue during a single breath-hold. The difference between this approach and the conventional approach is that the beam path trace for a single slice of tissue does not produce a planar section. A planar section is needed to satisfy the reconstruction algorithm. Therefore one more step is introduced in this process and that is *interpolation*. This is a part of the image reconstruction algorithms for MSCT technology, and it will be described in Chapter 15.

Multislice CT – essential principles: part 2

Figure 15.1 Examples of combining (binning) detector elements for the matrix array detector (a) and the adaptive array detector (b).

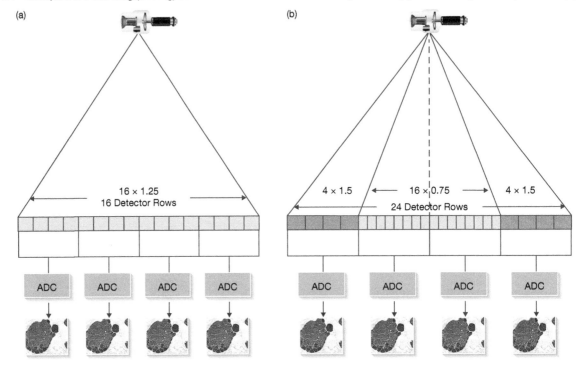

Figure 15.2 The effect of wide collimation (a) and narrow collimation (b) on the slice thickness and the visual image quality.

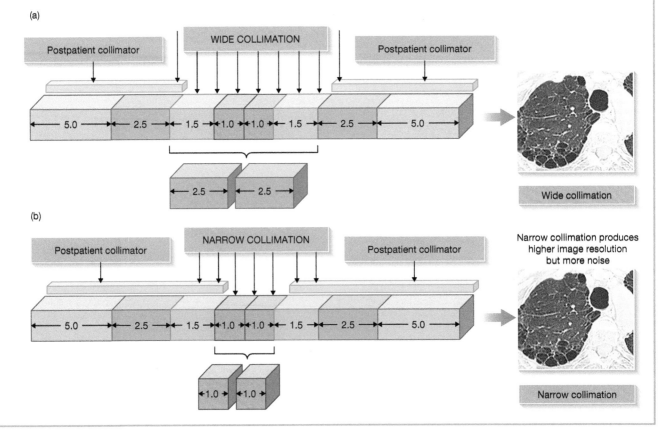

Figure 15.3 Effect of the interpolation technique on image quality in MSCT (a). Without interpolation, streak artifacts appear on the image (b). Interpolation gets rid of these artifacts (c).

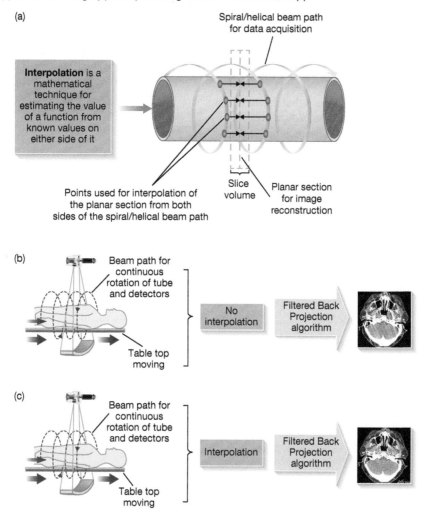

(a)

Spiral/helical beam path for data acquisition

Interpolation is a mathematical technique for estimating the value of a function from known values on either side of it

Points used for interpolation of the planar section from both sides of the spiral/helical beam path

Slice volume

Planar section for image reconstruction

(b)

Beam path for continuous rotation of tube and detectors

Table top moving

No interpolation

Filtered Back Projection algorithm

(c)

Beam path for continuous rotation of tube and detectors

Table top moving

Interpolation

Filtered Back Projection algorithm

Figure 15.4 Two types of interpolation approaches include 360° Z-interpolation (a) and 180° Z-interpolation (b).

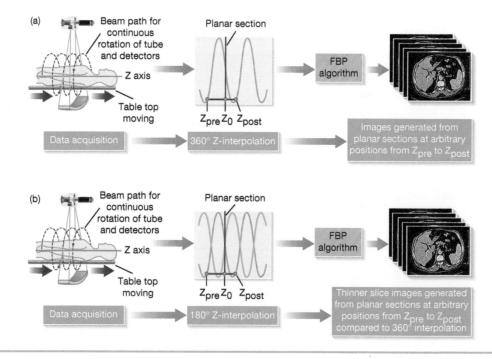

(a)

Beam path for continuous rotation of tube and detectors

Z axis

Table top moving

Planar section

Z_{pre} Z_0 Z_{post}

FBP algorithm

Data acquisition

360° Z-interpolation

Images generated from planar sections at arbitrary positions from Z_{pre} to Z_{post}

(b)

Beam path for continuous rotation of tube and detectors

Z axis

Table top moving

Planar section

Z_{pre} Z_0 Z_{post}

FBP algorithm

Data acquisition

180° Z-interpolation

Thinner slice images generated from planar sections at arbitrary positions from Z_{pre} to Z_{post} compared to 360° interpolation

Chapter 14 described the terminology and technical requirements for MSCT, including slip-ring technology, types of detectors, and data acquisition geometries for SSCT and MSCT. This chapter will deal specifically with detector configurations, effect of collimation on slice selection, image reconstruction, pitch, and selectable parameters.

MSCT detector configurations

The term *detector configuration* refers to the ways that the detector elements can be combined (binned) electronically to produce the desired slice thickness required for the examination, at the isocenter of the gantry. Figure 15.1 illustrates two examples of such binning for the matrix array detector (Figure 15.1a) and the adaptive array detector (Figure 15.1b). Each set of elements binned is coupled to an analog-to-digital converter (ADC) to produce the selected slices thickness (in both cases, four images are generated for each of the two detectors). Typical slice thicknesses that can be obtained include:

• 2 × 0.5 mm, 4 × 1.0 mm, 4 × 5.0 mm, 2 × 8.0 mm, and 2 × 10 mm for four-slice adaptive array detector;
• 16 × 0.5 mm, 16 × 1.0 mm, and 16 × 2.0 mm for a 16-slice matrix array detector.

Effect of collimation on slice thickness

In CT collimation defines the thickness of the slice of tissue to be imaged. Figure 15.2 illustrates the effect of wide collimation (Figure 15.2a) and narrow collimation (Figure 15.2b) on the slice thickness. Narrow collimation produces sharper images but more noise only if the exposure factors remain the same as an image produced by wider collimation.

Interpolation fundamentals

As described in Chapter 14 for SSCT, not all rays pass through the image plane (*planar section*) since the patient is moving through the gantry during scanning. Because of this an additional step of first calculating a planar section is required. This is done by interpolation, using data points on either side of the section. *Interpolation* is a mathematical procedure for estimating the value of a function from known values on either side of it, as shown in Figure 15.3. Without interpolation the images would demonstrate streaking artifacts, as shown in Figure 15.3b. Interpolation gets rid of these artifacts (Figure 15.3c)

Two types of interpolation approach include 360° Z-interpolation (Figure 15.4a) and 180° Z-interpolation (Figure 15.4b). The advantage of the latter is that thinner and sharper images can be produced compared to the former approach.

Iterative reconstruction algorithms (Chapter 10) are also now commonly used in modern day CT scanners.

Pitch

The International Electrotechnical Commission (IEC) defines MSCT *pitch* (P) = the distance the table travels per rotation (d)/ total collimation (W); that is, $P = d/W$. The total collimation, on the other hand, is equal to the number of slices (M) multiplied by the collimated slice thickness (S). Algebraically, the pitch can now be expressed as $P = d/W$ or $P = d/M \times S$. Two different pitch ratios are illustrated in Figure 15.5. The higher the pitch (Figure 15.5b), the faster the imaging time and the lower the dose to the patient; however, image quality will be poorer compared to a lower pitch (Figure 15.5a).

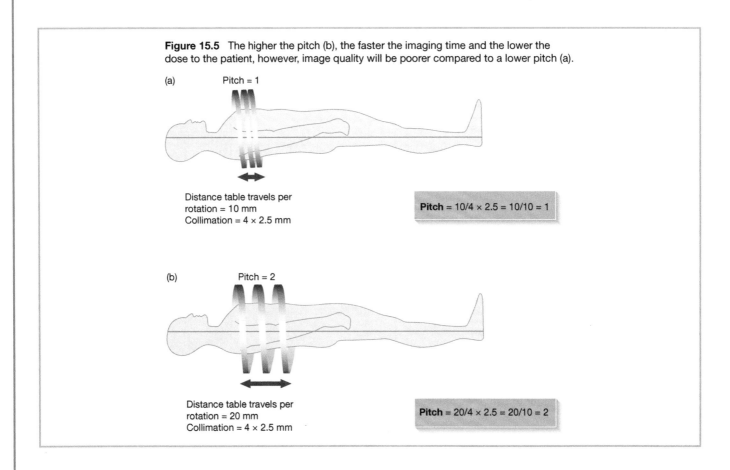

Figure 15.5 The higher the pitch (b), the faster the imaging time and the lower the dose to the patient, however, image quality will be poorer compared to a lower pitch (a).

(a) Pitch = 1

Distance table travels per rotation = 10 mm
Collimation = 4 × 2.5 mm

Pitch = 10/4 × 2.5 = 10/10 = 1

(b) Pitch = 2

Distance table travels per rotation = 20 mm
Collimation = 4 × 2.5 mm

Pitch = 20/4 × 2.5 = 20/10 = 2

Selectable parameters

MSCT offers the operator several selectable scan parameters to optimize not only the examination but also the dose to the patient. These parameters have been placed into two categories, namely *primary scan parameters* (PSPs) and *secondary reconstruction parameters* (SRPs). On the one hand, PSPs include tube current (mA), tube voltage (kVp), automatic exposure control (AEC), automatic voltage selection, pitch, scan time, and scan length. SRPs, on the other hand, include slice thickness, field of view (FOV), reconstruction algorithm, reconstruction interval, spatial resolution, contrast resolution, and geometric efficiency.

Dose optimization

The appropriate selection and control of the above parameters helps to ensure dose optimization. Optimization deals with reducing radiation dose while maintaining image quality; that is, using the lowest possible dose without compromising the diagnostic quality of the image. Dose reduction strategies, for example, relate to adjusting and controlling the technical factors affecting the dose with the goal of decreasing patient dose. The effect of these factors (e.g., mAs, kV, pitch, scan field-of-view, beam collimation, AEC, overbeaming and overranging, and iterative image reconstruction) on patient dose has been researched by multiple authors.

It is important that radiographers and radiologic technologists understand the distinction between CT dose reduction and CT dose optimization as well as the application of an "as low as reasonably achievable" (ALARA) philosophy of radiation protection, and remain active participants in optimizing patient dose and image quality in medical imaging, including CT.

16 Image quality: part 1

Figure 16.1 The quality of the CT image can be described by at least five physical parameters.

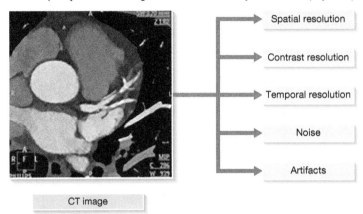

- Spatial resolution
- Contrast resolution
- Temporal resolution
- Noise
- Artifacts

CT image

Figure 16.2 Approximate spatial and contrast resolution values for radiographic and CT images.

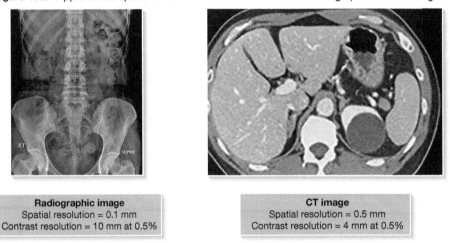

Radiographic image
Spatial resolution = 0.1 mm
Contrast resolution = 10 mm at 0.5%

CT image
Spatial resolution = 0.5 mm
Contrast resolution = 4 mm at 0.5%

Figure 16.3 Two CT phantoms for image quality assessment and quality control: the ACR GAMMEX 464 CT Accreditation Phantom (a) and the Cataphan® 700.
Source: (a) Gammex, Inc., Wisconsin, USA. Reproduced with permission of Gammex, Inc. (b) Reproduced with permission of The Phantom Laboratory, Incorporated.

Two popular CT phantoms

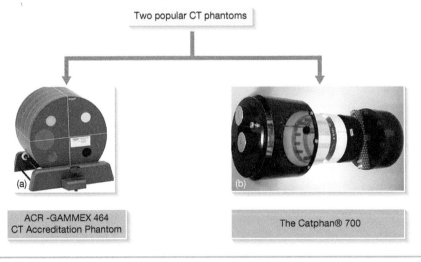

ACR -GAMMEX 464
CT Accreditation Phantom

The Catphan® 700

The CT image is a *digital image* and therefore image quality in CT is characterized by at least five physical factors shown in Figure 16.1, primarily spatial resolution, contrast resolution, temporal resolution, noise, and artifacts. The purpose of this chapter is to define and briefly outline methods for measuring each of them. In particular, two popular phantoms that are used to measure CT image quality will be described. Subsequent chapters will describe spatial, contrast, and temporal resolution; noise; and artifacts in detail.

Definitions

Spatial resolution is defined as the ability of the CT scanner to resolve closely spaced objects that are significantly different from their background, or the ability of the scanner to show small objects that have high subject contrast. The digital CT image is made up of a matrix of CT numbers, which must be converted into a gray-scale image for viewing by a human observer. There are at least *two major image quality objectives* in CT imaging; that is, to produce images that have high spatial resolution (sharp, high-detail images) and images with low noise. The degree of detail in this case depends on the matrix size, the field of view (FOV), and the slice thickness. Smaller pixel sizes for the same FOV will provide images with greater detail. The pixel size can be calculated using the following relationship: pixel size (p) = FOV/matrix size. Additionally thinner slice thicknesses will result in greater spatial sharpness of the image. Noise will be described later in the chapter. CT can show object sizes of 0.5 mm compared to 5 mm, 2 mm, 0.1 mm and 0.5 mm for nuclear medicine, diagnostic medical ultrasound (DMU), radiography, and magnetic resonance imaging (MRI), respectively. Radiography still offers the best spatial resolution of all the other imaging modalities, and hence is one

of the major reasons for its growth, development, and use in clinical practice.

Contrast resolution is the ability of the CT scanner to show small differences in soft tissues as demonstrated in Figure 16.2. While the radiographic image shows a contrast resolution (mm at 0.5%) of 10, the CT image shows a contrast resolution of 4, compared to 20 mm, 10 mm, 10 mm, and 1 mm for nuclear medicine, DMU, radiography, and magnetic resonance imaging, respectively. This simply means that CT has the advantage of showing soft tissues much better than radiography – one of the reasons for its continued development and use in clinical practice. MRI offers the best contrast resolution of all imaging modalities – a chief reason for its growth, development, and use in clinical practice.

Noise is the random variation of CT numbers in the image, and depends on not only the number of X-ray photons (*beam quantity*) falling on the image but also the beam energy (*beam quality*). Noise has a grainy or mottle appearance on the image. Larger voxels and thicker slices will result in more noise, compared with smaller voxels and thinner slices. Noise is described in detail in Chapter 19, since it is an important parameter not only for image quality but for radiation dose as well.

Temporal resolution is the ability of the scanner to freeze organ motion, such as the beating heart. It is an important parameter that deals in time or speed of acquiring data from the object, and is a required parameter when reducing motion is of primary consideration.

Artifacts are distortions or errors in the image that are not related to the object being imaged. They also include any discrepancy between the reconstructed CT image and the true attenuation coefficients of the object. Artifacts are described in more detail in Chapter 20.

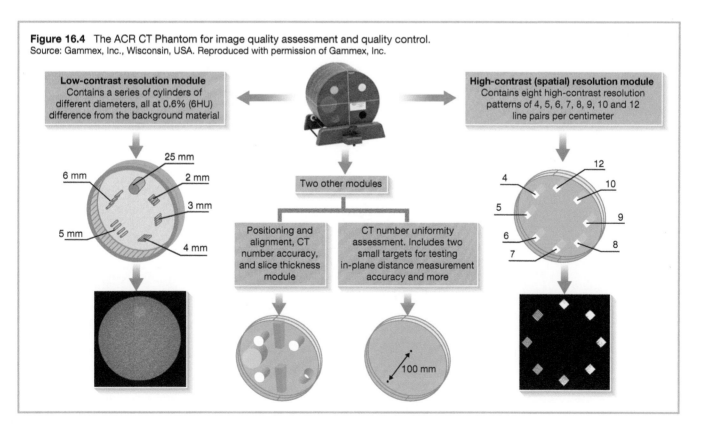

Figure 16.4 The ACR CT Phantom for image quality assessment and quality control.
Source: Gammex, Inc., Wisconsin, USA. Reproduced with permission of Gammex, Inc.

Low-contrast resolution module
Contains a series of cylinders of different diameters, all at 0.6% (6HU) difference from the background material

25 mm
6 mm
2 mm
3 mm
5 mm
4 mm

Two other modules

Positioning and alignment, CT number accuracy, and slice thickness module

CT number uniformity assessment. Includes two small targets for testing in-plane distance measurement accuracy and more

100 mm

High-contrast (spatial) resolution module
Contains eight high-contrast resolution patterns of 4, 5, 6, 7, 8, 9, 10 and 12 line pairs per centimeter

12
4
10
5
9
6
8
7

Phantoms for measuring CT image quality

Measurement of image quality parameters is vital not only for image quality assessment but also for CT quality control (QC). In this regard, there are several phantoms available for CT QC. Two such phantoms are shown in Figure 16.3. One of the most common phantoms is the *American College of Radiology (ACR) phantom*, and therefore a brief description is noteworthy here.

The phantom consists of four modules, as illustrated in Figure 16.4. While one module measures specifically spatial resolution, another module is designed to measure contrast resolution. A third module is used to assess CT number uniformity, and the fourth module is designed to address positioning and alignment issues, as well as CT number accuracy and slice thickness.

Image quality: part 2 – spatial resolution

Figure 17.1 Two elements of CT spatial resolution are the in-plane spatial resolution (X-Y axis image resolution) and the cross-plane spatial resolution (Z-axis image resolution).
Source: Reproduced with permission of The Phantom Laboratory, Incorporated.

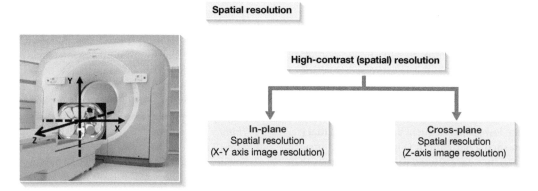

Figure 17.2 In-plane spatial resolution (X-Y image resolution) is expressed in line pairs per centimeter and spatial frequency (a). A typical bar pattern (b) and an image of the bar pattern (c) shown in (b).
Source: Reproduced with permission of The Phantom Laboratory, Incorporated.

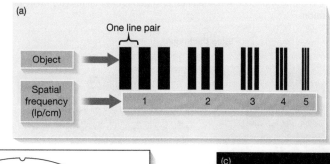

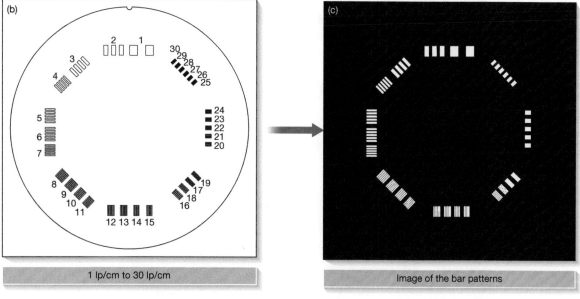

Figure 16.1 showed five image quality parameters, namely, spatial resolution, contrast resolution, temporal resolution, noise, and artifacts. The purpose of this chapter is to outline the factors affecting spatial resolution of the CT image. As defined in Chapter 16, *spatial resolution* is the ability of the CT scanner to resolve closely spaced objects that are significantly different from their background, or the ability of the scanner to show small objects that have high subject contrast. There are two elements of CT spatial resolution illustrated in Figure 17.1; the in-plane spatial resolution (X-Y axis image resolution) and the cross-plane spatial resolution (Z-axis image resolution).

In-plane spatial resolution

The *in-plane spatial resolution* measures the image resolution in the X-Y axis of the scanner, and it is expressed in terms of line pairs per centimeter (lp/cm) or in line pairs per millimeter (lp/mm). A line pair is defined as a bar (black) and a space (white) of equal size, as shown in Figure 17.2a. The series of bar patterns range from low spatial frequency (1) to high spatial frequency (5). When such a bar pattern (Figure 17.2b) is imaged by CT, the low-frequency bar patterns will appear sharper than the high-frequency patterns, as is clearly visible in Figure 17.2c.

While low spatial frequencies represent large objects, high frequencies represent small objects. In CT the spatial frequency is commonly expressed in lp/cm (Figure 17.2b) instead of lp/mm (for typical spatial resolution values of CT scanners refer to the vendors' technical specifications literature). In general, 10–14 lp/cm is possible in the standard CT imaging mode while 20 lp/cm is possible in the high-resolution imaging mode.

Factors affecting the in-plane spatial resolution

There are several factors affecting the in-plane spatial factors, including the slice thickness, detector cell size, collimation, reconstruction algorithm, pixel size and field of view (FOV), reconstruction filters, and other factors such as the focal spot size, scanner geometry, and so forth. It is not within the scope of this book to describe the details of how these factors affect spatial resolution; however, the following is noteworthy in helping the radiographer optimize image quality when scanning:

1 *Thinner slices* result in sharper images, as clearly visible in Figure 17.3a.
2 Smaller *detector sizes* will result in sharper images compared to larger sizes.

Figure 17.3 The effect of slice thickness (a) and convolution filters (b) on in-plane spatial resolution.

(a) Slice thickness — 10-mm — 1.5-mm

(b) Convolution filters — Standard kernel — Bone kernel

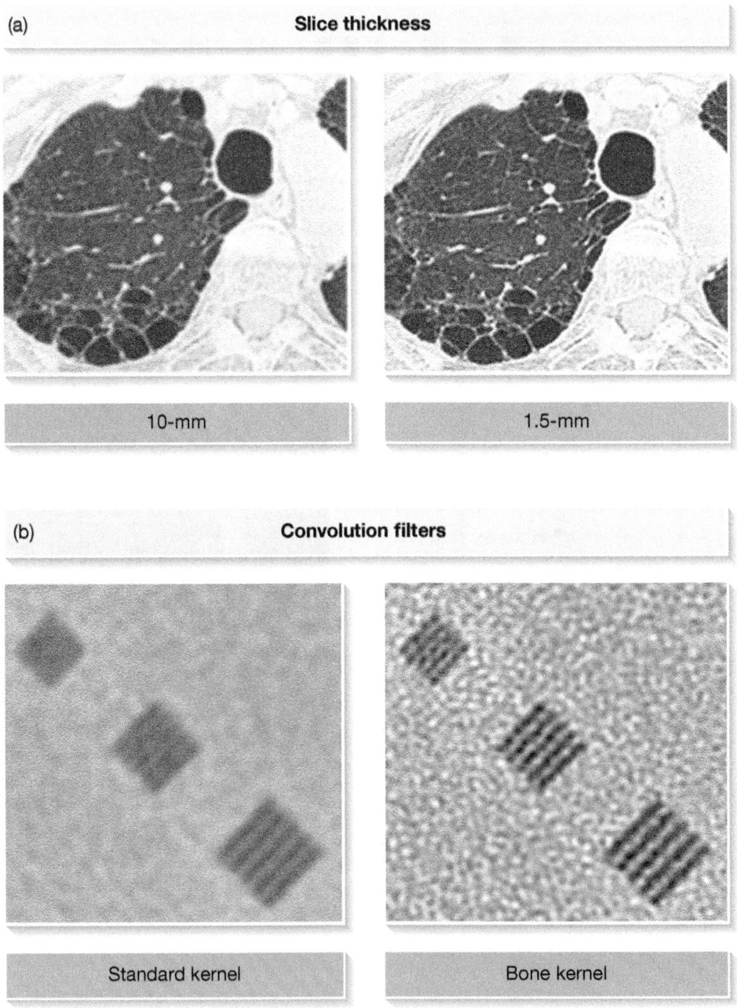

3 Smaller *focal spot sizes* will provide improved spatial resolution.

4 Narrow pre-detector *collimation* improves spatial resolution.

5 A *bone algorithm* produces a much sharper image than a standard algorithm (Figure 17.3b).

6 *Reconstruction algorithms* include the old Filtered Back Projection (FBP) algorithm, and the more recent reconstruction class of algorithms referred to as Iterative Reconstruction (IR) algorithms. An example of the effect of each of these two algorithms on the spatial resolution of the image is shown in Figure 10.4.

7 The *FOV* is related to the degree of sharpness that is required. Specifically, the reconstruction FOV is related to the pixel size as follows:

$$\text{Pixel size} = \text{FOV/Matrix size}$$

Smaller pixel sizes will show sharper images, for the same FOV.

Cross-plane spatial resolution

The *cross-plane spatial resolution* is the sharpness of the image that can be obtained along the Z-axis of the scanner. It is often described by the slice sensitivity profile (SSP), which is a plot of the beam intensity as a function of the location along the Z-axis (Figure 17.4). The slice thickness (hence the cross-plane resolution) can be obtained by measuring the full width at half maximum (FWHM) of the SSP curve. A noteworthy point, however, is that the FWHM is the distance between two points of the SSP curve with an intensity of 50% of the peak intensity. The SSP and FWHM are beyond the scope of this book.

The resolution in the Z-axis is much better with spiral/helical CT scanners compared with conventional CT scanners.

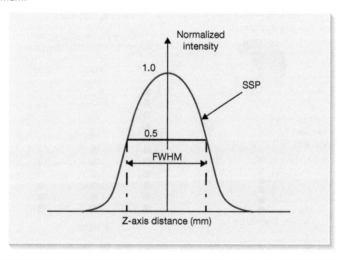

Figure 17.4 The cross-plane spatial resolution is the sharpness of the image that can be obtained along the Z-axis of the scanner. It is often described by the slice sensitivity profile (SSP), which is a plot of the beam intensity as a function of the location along the Z-axis. FWHM, full width at half maximum.

18 Image quality: part 3 – contrast resolution

Figure 18.1 Contrast resolution is the ability of the CT scanner to show low-contrast tissues whose density is slightly different from the background. For example, the soft tissues of fat and muscle are demonstrated very well in CT compared to radiography.

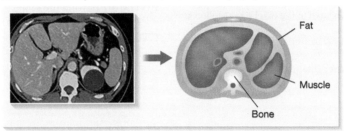

Figure 18.2 An illustration of contrast sensitivity.
Source: Courtesy of Dr Perry Sprawls PhD, Distinguished Emeritus Professor, Department of Radiology, Emory University School of Medicine, Atlanta, GA, USA.

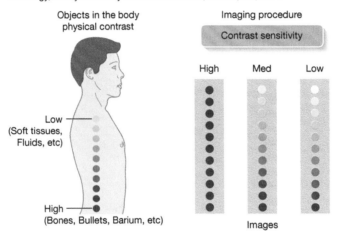

Figure 18.3   (a) A specially designed phantom for measuring contrast resolution, and (b) the image of this phantom.
Source: (b) Reproduced with permission of The Phantom Laboratory, Incorporated.

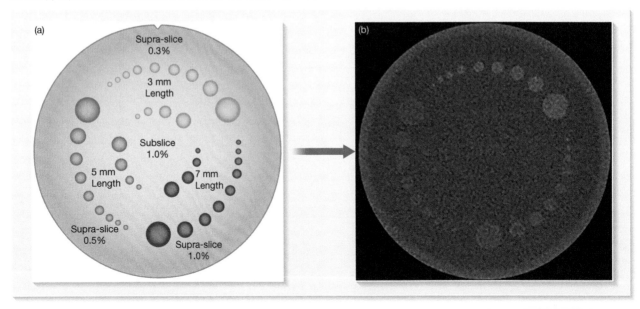

Figure 18.4 The visual appearance of low and high noise in phantom and patient images. High noise images appear very grainy.

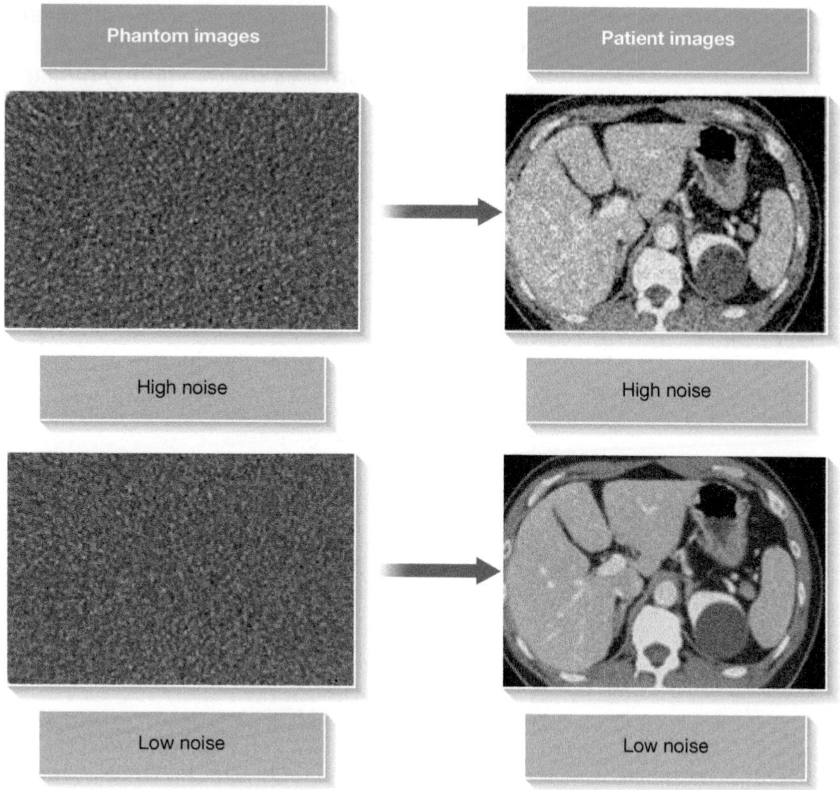

Definitions

Contrast resolution was defined in Chapter 16. In review it is the ability of the CT scanner to show low-contrast tissues whose density is slightly different from the background. For example, the soft tissues of fat and muscle are demonstrated very well in CT (Figure 18.1) compared to radiography. CT can detect density differences ranging from 0.25% to 0.5%, depending on the CT system.

The contrast resolution of an image in radiography is 10 mm at 0.5% while it is 4 mm at 0.5% in CT. Furthermore, this means that tissues such as fat and muscle, with small differences in not only atomic number but also mass density, will be clearly shown. These values are listed as follows:

Tissues	Atomic No. (Z)	Density (ρ)	CT Number
Bone	14	1.85	1000
Muscle	7.4	1.0	50
Fat	6.8	0.91	−100

Contrast sensitivity

The contrast resolution in CT is sometimes referred to as the sensitivity of the system or, more commonly, *contrast sensitivity*. This notion is clearly illustrated in Figure 18.2.

Low-contrast detectability

The low-contrast detectability (LCD), or low-contrast performance, of a CT scanner is typically defined as the smallest object that can be visualized at a given contrast level and dose.

Measurement of the contrast resolution

The contrast resolution in CT can be measured using specially designed phantoms. For example in Figure 18.3a, the low-contrast portion of the Catphan® (The Phantom Laboratory, Salem, New York, USA) is shown. There are three sets of disks with contrast of 0.3%, 0.5%, and 1.0%, and the sizes of the disks are 2 mm, 3 mm, 4 mm, 5 mm, 6 mm, 7 mm, 8 mm, 9 mm, and 15 mm. The image of this phantom is shown in Figure 18.3b. In CT, the contrast level is specified in terms of the percent linear attenuation coefficient. A 1% contrast means that the mean CT number of the object differs from its background by 10 HU. An important consideration to note in interpreting this image is that as the object size becomes smaller, it becomes increasingly difficult to identify a 0.3% contrast disk.

Factors affecting contrast resolution

The visibility of structures in the image is highly affected by noise, and there are several factors that influence the image noise (Figure 18.4). A few of them can be controlled by the operator and others are outside the operator's reach.

Factors under the operator's control include X-ray tube voltage (kV), tube current (mA), scan speed (sec), field of view (FOV), reconstruction algorithm selection, and slice thickness. Noise and the factors affecting it are highlighted in Chapter 19; however, the following points are noteworthy:

1 *Lower mA* results in fewer photons at the image receptor and hence results in an image with high noise (grainy image or an image showing increased mottle, as seen in Figure 18.4).

2 *Lower kV* results in fewer photons at the image receptor and hence in an image with high noise (grainy image or an image showing increased mottle – Figure 18.4).

3 As the *slice thickness* is increased, contrast resolution improves.
4 A *larger FOV* with a smaller matrix size (larger pixels) will result in improved contrast resolution.
5 The use of *iterative reconstruction (IR) algorithms* results in improved contrast resolution compared with the Filtered Back Projection (FBP) algorithm.

Temporal resolution

As noted by Dr Jiang Hsieh, chief medical physicist for a major CT manufacturer:

Temporal resolution is an indication of a CT system's ability to freeze motion of the scanned object. An oversimplified analogy is the "shutter" speed of a camera.

When a photo is taken at a sports event, a higher shutter speed should be used to reduce the blurring effects caused by the moving athletes. The awareness and importance of the temporal resolution for CT scanners has increased significantly in recent years thanks to an increased clinical utility of cardiac imaging. Because the heart motion is continuous and often irregular, cardiac imaging is one of the most challenging clinical applications for CT.

A major factor affecting temporal resolution is scan speed. By increasing the scan speed, the scanner has the ability to freeze the motion of objects (e.g., the beating heart), which will result in sharper images.

19 Image quality: part 4 – noise

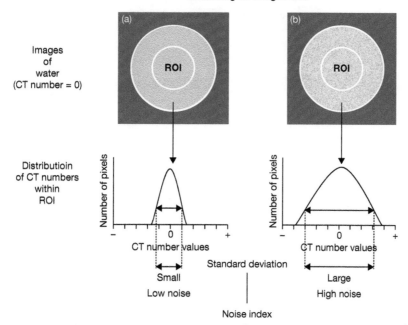

Figure 19.1 Noise can range from high to low. High noise limits the number of objects that can be seen.
Source: Courtesy of Dr Perry Sprawls PhD, Distinguished Emeritus Professor, Department of Radiology, Emory University School of Medicine, Atlanta, GA, USA.

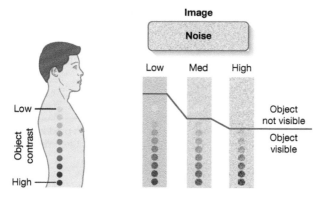

Figure 19.2 Schematic illustration of how to measure CT image noise. While image (a) has less noise and smaller SD, image (b) has high noise and a greater SD.
Source: Courtesy of Dr Perry Sprawls PhD, Distinguished Emeritus Professor, Department of Radiology, Emory University School of Medicine, Atlanta, GA, USA.

CT at a Glance, First Edition. Euclid Seeram.
© 2018 John Wiley & Sons, Ltd. Published 2018 by John Wiley & Sons, Ltd.

Definition

Noise was first defined in Chapter 16, and subsequently mentioned in Chapter 17, where it was shown that contrast resolution is limited by image noise. Recall that the CT image is a digital image made up of numbers, CT numbers that represent attenuation values in the patient. In review *noise* is defined as the random variation of CT numbers in the image, and depends on not only the mA (*beam quantity*) but also the kV (*beam quality*). Noise can range from high to low, as illustrated in Figure 19.1, which shows that high noise limits the number of objects that can be seen. In fact, a large variation of CT numbers in the image of a water bath means that the image is very noisy. If all pixel values were equal the noise in the image would be zero.

Phantom measurement of the noise

A water phantom of approximately 20 cm in diameter is generally used to measure CT image noise. Once the image of the phantom is obtained, the operator defines a region of interest (ROI) on the image and the CT numbers are plotted as a function of the number of pixels in the ROI. Subsequently, the standard deviation (SD), which is a measure of the noise in the ROI, is calculated. Figure 19.2 illustrates this with two images (a) and (b).

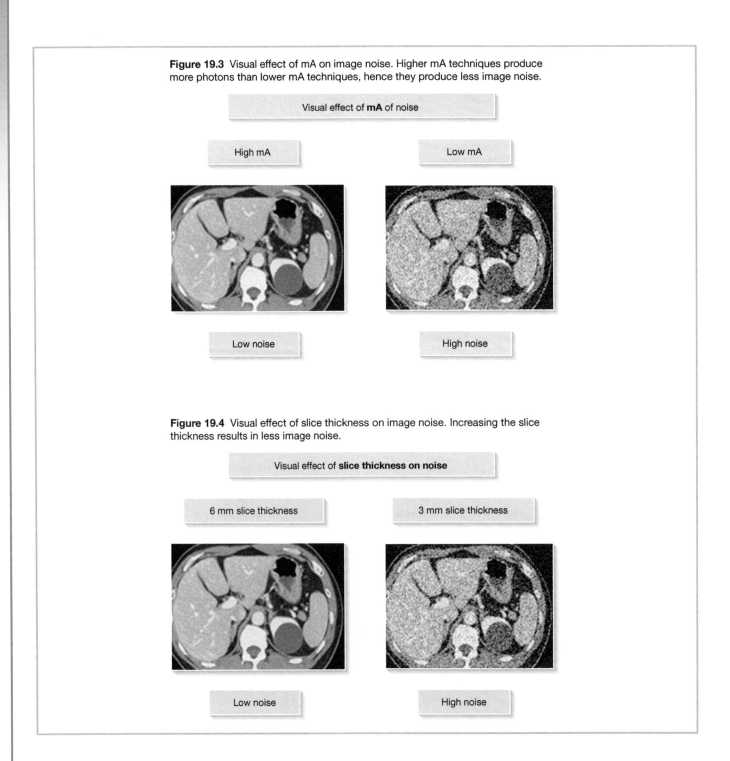

Figure 19.3 Visual effect of mA on image noise. Higher mA techniques produce more photons than lower mA techniques, hence they produce less image noise.

Visual effect of **mA** of noise

High mA

Low mA

Low noise

High noise

Figure 19.4 Visual effect of slice thickness on image noise. Increasing the slice thickness results in less image noise.

Visual effect of **slice thickness on noise**

6 mm slice thickness

3 mm slice thickness

Low noise

High noise

While image (a) has less noise and smaller SD, image (b) has high noise and a greater SD.

Factors affecting noise

There are several factors affecting CT image noise. These include kV, mA, filtration, pixel size, slice thickness, detector efficiency, algorithm, and patient dose. The following points are important in controlling image noise:

1 Higher *kV* techniques produce more photons than lower kV techniques, hence less image noise.

2 Higher *mA* techniques produce more photons than lower mA techniques, hence less image noise, as shown in Figure 19.3.

3 Greater *beam filtration* reduces the number of photons at the detector, resulting in more image noise.

4 Increasing *slice thickness* results in less image noise, as shown in Figure 19.4.

5 Increasing *pixel size* creates less image noise.

6 Higher *detector efficiency* captures more photons and therefore will result in less image noise.

7 *Iterative reconstruction (IR) algorithms* will produce images with less noise compared to the Filtered Back Projection (FBP) reconstruction algorithm.

8 High *radiation doses* result in less image noise, and better images; however, operators are committed to work within the As Low As Reasonably Achievable (ALARA) philosophy in terms of radiation protection of the patient.

One of the major goals of imaging patients with the CT scanner is to optimize the dose. This means that operators must ensure that low doses are used but image quality must not be compromised. Such consideration leads to the notion of *dose optimization*, an increasingly important element in CT. This will be discussed in Chapters 21 and 22.

20 Image quality: part 5 – artifacts

Figure 20.1 A classification of CT artifacts shown not only as graphic appearances but also how they appear on images.
Source: Courtesy of Jiang Hsieh PhD, Chief Scientist, Applied Science Lab, General Electric Healthcare Technologies, Waukesha, WI, USA.

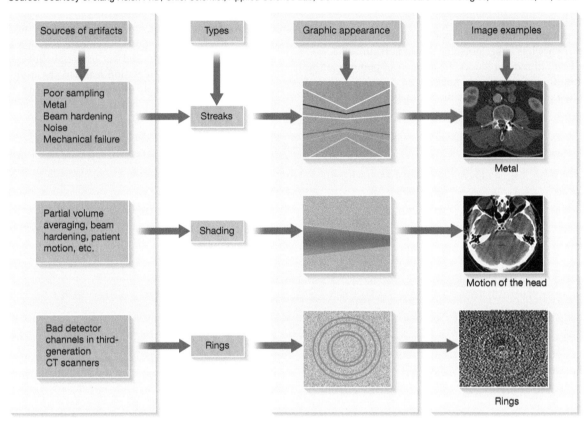

Figure 20.2 Patient motion creates streaks on the image (a), which can be corrected (b) using the appropriate software.
Source: Courtesy of Jiang Hsieh PhD, Chief Scientist, Applied Science Lab, General Electric Healthcare Technologies, Waukesha, WI, USA.

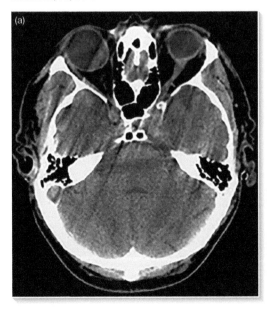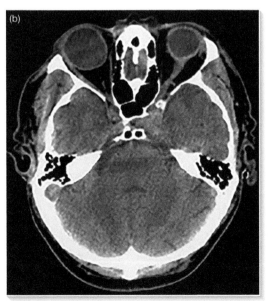

CT at a Glance, First Edition. Euclid Seeram.
© 2018 John Wiley & Sons, Ltd. Published 2018 by John Wiley & Sons, Ltd.

Definition

Artifacts in CT can cause confusion for radiologists during image interpretation because they appear on images but are not present on or in the patient. In 1995 Dr Jiang Hsieh, a senior medical physicist with a major CT manufacturer, defined an artifact as "any discrepancy between the reconstructed CT numbers in the image and the true attenuation coefficients of the object." Dr Hsieh emphasized that the definition "implies that anything that causes an incorrect measurement of transmission readings by the detectors or an inconsistency between the measurement and reconstruction will result in an image artefact."

Types of artifacts

A classification of CT artifacts is shown in Figure 20.1. Such classification is based on how the artifacts appear on the image. These artifacts can appear as *streaks*, *bands of shading*, *rings and other appearances* such as *moiré patterns*, and *basket weave*. Furthermore, Figure 20.1 shows not only graphic appearances but also how the artifacts appear on images. It is important for

Figure 20.3 Beam hardening artifact, which appears as shading differences on the image (a), while (b) shows the correction of the artifact.
Source: Courtesy of Jiang Hsieh PhD, Chief Scientist, Applied Science Lab, General Electric Healthcare Technologies, Waukesha, WI, USA.

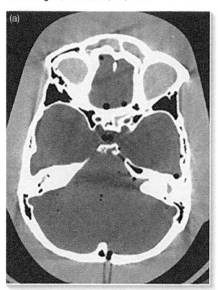 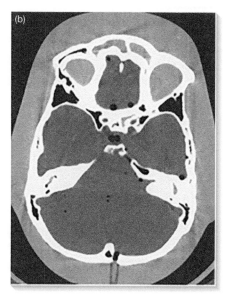

Figure 20.4 Artifacts from partial volume averaging. In (a) a 7-mm detector aperture was used while in (b) a 1-mm detector aperture was used to minimize this artifact.
Source: Courtesy of Jiang Hsieh PhD, Chief Scientist, Applied Science Lab, General Electric Healthcare Technologies, Waukesha, WI, USA.

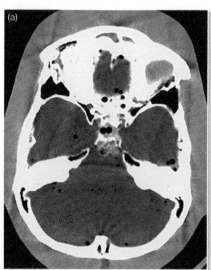 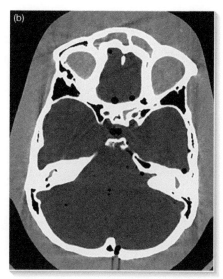

radiologists and radiographers to be able to identify these artifacts in an effort to improve diagnosis.

Causes of artifacts

There are several causes of the above mentioned artifacts and these are listed in Figure 20.1 as well. They include: poor sampling, partial volume averaging, metal, beam hardening, noise, mechanical failure, patient motion, and bad detector channels in third-generation CT scanners.

Common artifacts

It is not within the scope of this book to describe the above artifacts in any detail; however, the more common ones arise from patient motion, the presence of metal in or on the patient, beam hardening, and partial volume averaging. The following points provide a generalized overview of:

1 *Patient motion* is usually involuntary or voluntary and this will create streaks on the image. An example is shown in Figure 20.2a. These streaks can be corrected by software (Figure 20.2b) and by providing clear instructions to the patient about the need for appropriate breathing and the essential need not to move during the scanning procedure.

2 *Beam hardening* refers to an increase in the mean energy of the X-ray beam as it passes through the patient. This phenomenon leads to the creating of artifacts that appear as shading differences on the image, as shown in Figure 20.3a, while Figure 20.3b shows the correction of the artifact.

3 The presence of *metal*, such as surgical clips, prostheses, or dental fillings, creates streaking artifacts. The metal absorbs more radiation than the surrounding tissues and this results in a loss of information in the projection profiles from the detectors, leading to streaks on the image.

4 *Partial volume averaging* occurs when a voxel contains more than one tissue type. For example, if a voxel contains three different tissue types, such as bone, soft tissue, and air, the CT number computed will be an average of the three tissues. This phenomenon leads to shading differences referred to as partial volume averaging artifacts, as shown in Figure 20.4a. These artifacts can be corrected using thinner slices, for example, as shown in Figure 20.4b.

As noted earlier in this chapter, artifacts in CT can arise from several sources. These artifacts are based on the physics of CT imaging, the CT scanner itself, and the patient. It is important that both radiologists and radiographers are able to recognize these artifacts and make every effort to correct them by always using the appropriate measures.

21 CT dose optimization: part 1

Figure 21.1 Two categories of dose-response models used in medical imaging. (a) A linear dose-response model without a threshold (LNT) and (b) a linear dose-response model with a threshold.

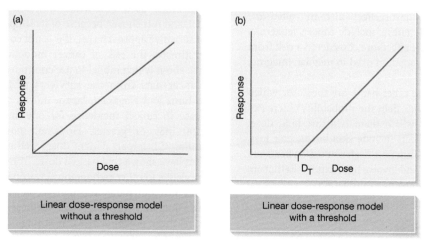

(a)
Response
Dose
Linear dose-response model
without a threshold

(b)
Response
D_T Dose
Linear dose-response model
with a threshold

Figure 21.2 The typical dose distribution $D(z)$ is a bell-shaped curve (a). Typical phantoms, a head phantom (b) and a body phantom (c), used to measure $D(z)$. A pencil ionization chamber is used to capture the radiation and is positioned as shown in (c).

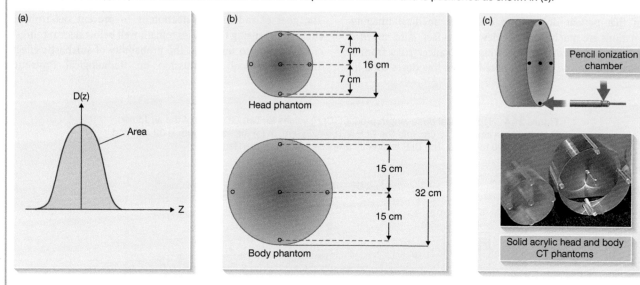

(a)
$D(z)$
Area
Z

(b)
7 cm
16 cm
7 cm
Head phantom

15 cm
32 cm
15 cm
Body phantom

(c)
Pencil ionization chamber
Solid acrylic head and body CT phantoms

Figure 21.3 The equations used to calculate three dose metrics used in CT. See text for further explanation.

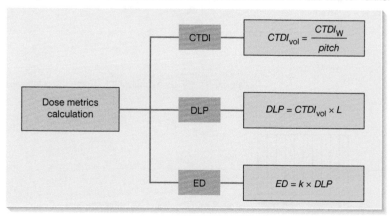

Dose metrics calculation

CTDI
$$CTDI_{vol} = \frac{CTDI_W}{pitch}$$

DLP
$$DLP = CTDI_{vol} \times L$$

ED
$$ED = k \times DLP$$

CT at a Glance, First Edition. Euclid Seeram.
© 2018 John Wiley & Sons, Ltd. Published 2018 by John Wiley & Sons, Ltd.

Risks of radiation exposure

Radiation protection guides, recommendations, and standards and are based on the knowledge of the *biological effects of radiation exposure*. These effects fall into two broad categories, namely stochastic effects and deterministic effects. *Stochastic effects* are random, and the probability of their occurrence depends on the amount of radiation dose an individual receives. The probability increases as the dose increases, and there is no threshold dose for stochastic effects. These effects become apparent years after exposure; therefore, stochastic effects also are called *late effects*. Examples of stochastic effects include cancer, leukemia, and genetic damage. Stochastic effects are considered a risk from exposure to the low levels of radiation used in medical imaging, including CT examinations.

Deterministic effects on the other hand, are those for which the severity of the effect (rather than the probability) increases with radiation dose and for which there is a threshold dose. Examples of deterministic effects include skin burns, hair loss, tissue damage, and organ dysfunction. Deterministic effects are also referred to as *early effects* and involve high exposures that are unlikely to occur in medical imaging examinations.

Dose-response models

It has been shown by the Radiation Effects Research Foundation that at high doses (100 mSv [millisievert] and higher), the evidence of increased cancer is statistically significant. It is well known that patient doses from diagnostic medical imaging examinations are much lower. In view of this fact, *dose-response models* have been proposed to extrapolate cancer risks from a high-dose situation to the risks posed by the low doses used in diagnostic imaging. These models fall into two categories: a linear dose-response model without a threshold (LNT) (Figure 21.1a) and a linear dose-response model with a threshold (Figure 21.1b). While the former model shows that no amount of radiation is considered safe and that any dose, no matter how small, carries some degree of risk, the latter proposes that no adverse effect from radiation below a certain level (the threshold dose = D_T) is observed. A biological response is observed only when the threshold dose is reached.

The model used most widely in medical imaging is the LNT model, and it is chosen because of its simplicity and because it is a conservative approach (i.e., if it is not correct, then it probably overestimates the risk of cancer induction at low dose). The debate about which model to use continues.

Cancer data from the survivors of the atomic bombs at Hiroshima and Nagasaki, Japan, show a statistically significant increase in cancer incidence for one-time acute exposure of 50–100 mSv or greater. However, most diagnostic exams, including CT, impart patient doses well below 20 mSv. Several studies have shown that patient doses from CT examinations are high relative to other radiography examinations. For example, as of 2011, CT contributed the highest collective dose in the United States compared with any other medical imaging modality. In view of these potential risks, it is mandatory for the imaging community to protect patients.

Radiation protection philosophy

The goal of radiation protection is to prevent deterministic effects by ensuring that doses remain well below relevant threshold doses and to minimize the probability of stochastic effects. The International Commission on Radiological Protection

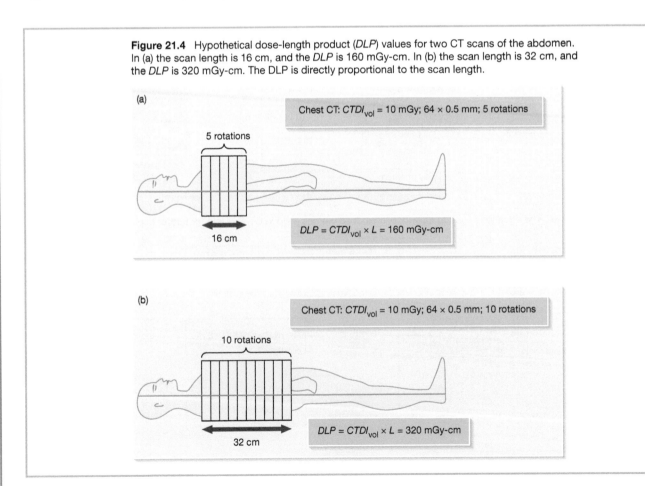

Figure 21.4 Hypothetical dose-length product (*DLP*) values for two CT scans of the abdomen. In (a) the scan length is 16 cm, and the *DLP* is 160 mGy-cm. In (b) the scan length is 32 cm, and the *DLP* is 320 mGy-cm. The DLP is directly proportional to the scan length.

(a)

Chest CT: $CTDI_{vol}$ = 10 mGy; 64 × 0.5 mm; 5 rotations

5 rotations

16 cm

$DLP = CTDI_{vol} \times L = 160$ mGy-cm

(b)

Chest CT: $CTDI_{vol}$ = 10 mGy; 64 × 0.5 mm; 10 rotations

10 rotations

32 cm

$DLP = CTDI_{vol} \times L = 320$ mGy-cm

(ICRP) offers three fundamental principles that guide in protecting patients. These include justification, optimization, and the application of dose limits. While principles of justification and optimization address individuals who are exposed to radiation, and the principle of dose limits deals with occupational and environmental exposures and excludes medical exposure, the principle of optimization is intended to protect the patient from unnecessary radiation by using a dose that is As Low As Reasonably Achievable (ALARA). The ultimate goal of optimization is to minimize stochastic effects and to prevent deterministic effects. Optimization will be described in detail in Chapter 22.

CT dose measurement

The typical dose distribution is a bell-shaped curve, as shown in Figure 21.2a. The dose distribution is given by the function $D(z)$, where D is the dose and z is the longitudinal axis of the patient. $D(z)$ is extremely important to the CT dose because this is the dose distribution, or dose profile, which is measured. Typical phantoms used to measure $D(z)$ are shown in Figure 21.2b and c.

Dose metrics use in CT

At least three dose metrics are displayed on the CT scanner after each examination. These include the *computed tomography dose index* (*CTDI*) and the *dose-length product* (*DLP*), and the *effective dose* (*ED*). The CT dose index (CTDI) is a standardized measure of radiation dose output of a CT scanner that allows the user to compare radiation outputs of different CT scanners. It provides a measurement of the exposure per slice, and information about the amount of radiation used to perform the study. CT vendors are required to provide $CTDI_{vol}$ values on the CT scanner console. The equations used to calculate the three dose metrics are shown in Figure 21.3.

The value of the $CTDI_{vol}$ is the same whether a technologist scans a 1-mm or 100-mm length of tissue. The *DLP* was introduced to provide a much more accurate representation of the dose for a defined length of tissue. The *DLP* provides a measure of the total dose for a CT (*L* equals the length of the scan (in centimeters) along the patient's *z*-axis. *DLP* is expressed in mGy-cm. Although the $CTDI_{vol}$ does not depend on scan length, the *DLP* is directly proportional to the scan length. This is illustrated in Figure 21.4.

Finally the *ED* allows one to compare the dose received from CT with the dose received from natural background radiation. For example, while the annual effective dose from natural background radiation is reported to be 3 mSv, it is 2.0 mSv for CT of the head, and 10 mSv for CT of the abdomen and pelvis.

22 CT dose optimization: part 2

Figure 22.1 The difference between overbeaming and overranging in CT. Adaptive or dynamic collimation also is illustrated.
Source: Goo HW. CT radiation dose optimization and estimation: an update for radiologists, *Korean J Radiology* 2012;13(1):1–11. Reproduced with permission of the *Korean Journal of Radiology*, the Korean Society of Radiology.

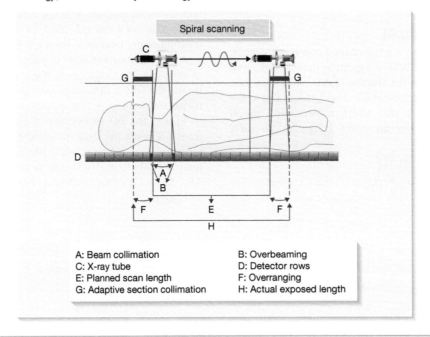

A: Beam collimation B: Overbeaming
C: X-ray tube D: Detector rows
E: Planned scan length F: Overranging
G: Adaptive section collimation H: Actual exposed length

Factors affecting the dose in CT

Several surveys on patient doses in CT in different countries have shown a downward trend in average effective dose (mSv) due to technical and physics-based improvements in the CT scanner, as well as dose optimization efforts on the part of the user.

There are several factors affecting dose in CT, and optimization methods emphasize that dose and image quality go "hand-in-hand." This means that using the lowest possible dose (to keep within the ALARA philosophy) must not compromise the diagnostic quality of the image.

In general a mathematical expression that relates dose and several image quality factors is:

$$\text{Dose} = k \times \frac{\text{Intensity} \times \text{Beam energy}}{\text{Noise}^2 \times \text{Pixel size}^3 \times \text{Slice thickness}}$$

where k is a conversion factor. Furthermore, this expression implies the following practical points for the radiographer:

1 *Increasing milliamperage* (intensity) and *kilovoltage* (beam energy) increases patient dose proportionally. For example, while a two-fold increase in milliamperage increases the dose by a factor of two, doubling the dose requires an increase by the square of the kilovolt peak.

2 Reducing the *noise* in an image by a factor of two requires an increase in the dose by a factor of four.

3 Improving the spatial resolution (*pixel size*) by a factor of two requires an increase in the dose by a factor of eight.

4 Decreasing the *slice thickness* by a factor of two requires an increase in the dose by a factor of two (keeping the noise constant).

5 Decreasing both *slice thickness and pixel size* (spatial resolution) by a factor of two requires an increase in the dose by a factor of 16 ($2^3 \times 2 = 2 \times 2 \times 2 \times 2$).

There are *other important factors with spiral/helical CT scanners* such as the pitch, effective mAs, and other technical developments with the main goal of higher dose efficiency. Specifically, these include automatic exposure control (tube current modulation), automatic voltage selection (X-ray spectra optimization), X-ray beam collimation, more efficient X-ray detectors, and iterative reconstruction algorithms.

Pitch

The pitch is defined by the International Electrotechnical Commission (IEC) as a ratio of the distance the table travels per rotation to the total collimated X-ray beam width. The dose is inversely proportional to the pitch.

Effective mAs

The effective mAs is the product of the tube current and the exposure time (true mAs) per rotation divided by the pitch.

Automatic exposure control (AEC)

The goal of AEC, specifically automatic tube current modulation (ATCM), is to adjust the mA in either the *z*-axis (longitudinal), the *x-y*-axis (angular), or both, in an effort to reduce patient dose. The literature suggests that ATCM has a dose reduction potential from about 10% to 60%.

Automatic tube voltage selection

When using automatic voltage selection the AEC selects the optimal tube potential (to optimize the X-ray spectra) according to the diagnostic task and patient size in order to achieve the desired image quality at a lower $CTDI_{vol}$. It is important to note that the kV is not modulated in the same manner as mA (ATCM) and does not change with tube positions around the patient; however, the kV is held constant for the diagnostic task at hand, but can change for a different diagnostic task. Furthermore, when changing the kV, the mA needs to be adapted as well to maintain a constant contrast-to-noise ratio. The literature shows this technique has a dose reduction potential from about 10% to 50%.

Adaptive beam collimation

Adaptive collimation is used in modern CT scanners to reduce patient dose at the beginning and end of scanning to address issues with overranging and overbeaming.

While *overranging* refers to the use of additional rotations before and after the planned length of tissue so the first and last images can be reconstructed, *overbeaming* is the excess dose beyond the edge of the detector rows per rotation of a multisection (Figure 22.1). Both overranging and overbeaming increase radiation dose to the patient. The literature suggests that adaptive collimation has a dose reduction potential ranging from about 5% to 40%.

Iterative reconstruction (IR) algorithms

Important advantages of iterative image reconstruction algorithms are to reduce image noise and minimize the higher radiation dose inherent in the Filtered Back Projection algorithm. Several studies have demonstrated that IR algorithms have a dose reduction potential ranging from about 10% to 60%

More efficient CT detectors

Improvements to CT detectors – most notably using directly converting sensors such as cadmium telluride, miniaturization of the electronics in the data acquisition system (DAS) using nanotechnology, and electronic noise reduction – have led to scanning with lower tube outputs. The literature shows that these detectors have a dose reduction potential from about 10% to 40%.

Optimization of radiation protection in CT

Several methods and processes for effective radiation protection of the patient involve at least four elements, as follows:

1 Dose optimization methods.

2 Regulatory and guidance recommendations for imaging facilities and personnel.

3 Diagnostic reference levels.

4 Campaigns to promote radiation awareness and safety in CT.

5 CT dose optimization responsibilities.

These will be described briefly in Chapter 23.

23 Optimization of radiation protection in CT

Figure 23.1 A common methodology for effective optimization of radiation protection in CT.

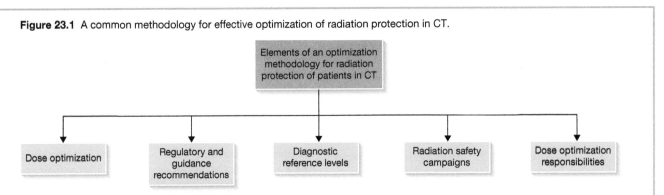

Figure 23.2 Mean dose from an AP pelvis arranged in increasing magnitude. The horizontal line at the third quartile value represents the DRL of 8 mGy.

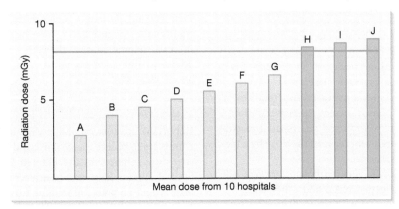

Table 23.1 An example of an optimization checklist in CT. This is a useful first tool in the radiation protection optimization methodology. Source: Goo HW. CT radiation dose optimization and estimation: an update for radiologists, *Korean J Radiology* 2012;13(1):1–11. Reproduced with permission of the *Korean Journal of Radiology*, the Korean Society of Radiology.

Checkup items	Recommendations
Body size-adapted CT protocol	√ Traditionally based on body weight or body mass index √ Based on cross-sectional dimensions and/or body attenuation for better dose adaptation to individually varied body habitus √ Use best-fit equation rather than dose table or chart
Tube current modulation	√ Always turn on if applicable √ Set up appropriate reference image quality index √ Check how much modulated tube current reaches to maximal limits ("tube current saturation") and adjust parameters such as tube voltage and scan speed to obtain maximal dose reduction by tube current modulation
Optimal tube voltage at equivalent radiation dose	√ Select most dose-efficient tube voltage √ Consider lower tube voltages for contrast-enhanced examination, higher tube voltages for examinations requiring lower noise (e.g., unenhanced brain CT) and for examinations detecting low-contrast lesions (e.g., microabscesses in liver or ground-glass opacity in lung)
Longitudinal scan range	√ Adjust to minimal range as required for clinical indications, desirably by using clear anatomic landmarks
Repeated scanning	√ Reduce number of repeated scanning √ Omit precontrast examination if possible
Scan modes	√ Use low-dose scan mode to maximize benefit-risk ratio of CT examination (e.g., prospectively ECG-triggered sequential or high-pitch dual-source spiral scanning in cardiac CT)
Noise-reducing image reconstruction algorithms	√ Use noise-reducing, spatial resolution-preserving algorithms (e.g., iterative reconstruction algorithms) at lower radiation dose

Table 23.2 Examples of specific reports addressing CT radiation protection regulatory and guidance.

Organization	Examples of reports
ICRP	ICRP Publication 102: Managing Patient Dose in Multi-Detector Computed Tomography (MDCT). *Ann ICRP* 2007; 37 (1)
NRPB-PHE	Protection of the Patient in X-ray Computed Tomography. *NRPB* Vol. 3, No. 4 (2013)
US FDA	CFR-Code of Federal Regulations-Title 21: Sec. 1020.33-Performance Standards for Ionizing Radiation Emitting Products: Computed Tomography (CT) equipment (2016)
Health Canada	Safety Code 35 (SC 35) Radiation Protection in Radiology-Large Facilities; Section 2.5.4: Computed Tomography Equipment Requirements

Optimization methodologies

When discussing how closely to follow the ALARA principle and balance the need for patient radiation protection with the need for acquiring high-quality diagnostic images, the literature most often uses two terms: reduction and optimization. While *reduction* means to "reduce or diminish in size, amount, extent, or number," *optimization* means "an act, process, or methodology of making something (as a design, system, or decision) as fully perfect, functional, or effective as possible."

Several articles in the literature have described various strategies for dose reduction and deal with how to adjust and control the technical factors (e.g., mAs, kVp, pitch, scan field of view, beam collimation, AEC, and iterative image reconstruction) affecting the dose with the goal of decreasing patient dose (see Chapter 22). Dose optimization, on the other hand, based on image quality (e.g., high-contrast spatial resolution, low-contrast resolution, temporal resolution, noise, and artifacts), requires a thorough understanding of CT dose metrics (see Chapter 21) and CT image quality parameters (see Chapter 16).

A common methodology for effective optimization of radiation protection in CT is illustrated in Figure 23.1. This includes a dose optimization checklist, regulatory and guidance recommendations, diagnostic reference levels, radiation safety campaigns, and dose optimization responsibilities. Each of these will be described briefly below.

Dose optimization checklist

The establishment and use of an optimization checklist in CT is a useful first tool in the radiation protection optimization methodology. Several recommended lists have been identified in the literature. An example of one such recommended checklist is shown in Table 23.1, which identifies seven elements common to most of the other lists in the literature. Of these it is important to pay attention to items that are common to CT protocols, such as the tube current modulation, tube voltage selection, low-dose scan modes, and iterative reconstruction algorithms.

Regulatory and guidance recommendations

Radiation protection of patients, including CT, is an important issue addressed by several organizations at international and national levels. Among these are the International Commission on Radiological Protection (ICRP), the National Radiation Protection Board (NRPB) – which became the Radiation Protection Division of the Health Protection Agency (HPA), now a part of Public Health England (PHE) – the United States Food and Drug Administration (FDA), and Health Canada. Table 23.2 provides examples of specific reports addressing CT radiation protection regulatory and guidance recommendations. Furthermore, these regulations also feature comprehensive recommendations and guidance on quality control of CT scanners (described in Chapter 24). Users should consult the appropriate report related to their respective countries.

Diagnostic reference levels

The term diagnostic reference level (DRL) was first introduced in 1996 by the ICRP, and used to optimize dose levels and image quality; it represents yet another method of optimizing radiation protection of patients in CT. A DRL is defined as an *investigational level used to identify unusually high radiation doses* for common diagnostic examinations.

In Figure 23.2, the mean dose for an AP pelvis from 10 hospitals is shown. The DRL represents the third quartile value, which corresponds to 8 mGy. Note that three hospitals exceed this value. This means that those three hospitals should pay close attention to their radiation protection of the patient to bring their levels at or below the DRL. The American College of Radiology (ACR), for example, recommends that the DRL for an adult abdomen and pelvis, and adult chest should be 25 mGy and 21 mGy, respectively.

Radiation safety campaigns

There are several campaigns to promote radiation awareness and safety worldwide. Two popular campaigns include "Image Gently" (www.imagegently.org) and "Image Wisely" (http://www.imagewisely.org). While the former is intended to have an impact on practice by raising awareness to reduce radiation dose in pediatric imaging including CT, the latter focuses on resources and information on radiation safety in adult medical imaging, including CT. Both of these campaigns are supported by several radiology and physics organizations including the ACR, and the American Association of Physicists in Medicine (AAPM), for example. Furthermore, in Europe, the campaign is called "EuroSafe," and it is intended to "promote radiation protection and safety and provide information to make informed decisions regarding imaging."

CT dose optimization responsibilities

When considering radiation protection optimization in CT, it is important that imaging facilities assign responsibilities to specific individuals whose efforts should focus on various actions (as described in an article entitled CT Radiation Dose Management by Dr Anushri Parakh and others published in *Radiology* in 2016). These actions include *dose justification*, *dose optimization*, and *dose management*. While referring physicians and radiologists assume responsibility for the first action, radiographers, radiologists, and medical physicists assume responsibilities for the second and third actions.

Justification would occur before the CT examination and would involve risk-benefit analysis; optimization would occur during the CT scanning and would focus attention on the use of the lowest dose possible; and dose management would occur after the CT examination and its major focus would be centered around dose tracking.

24 CT quality control basics

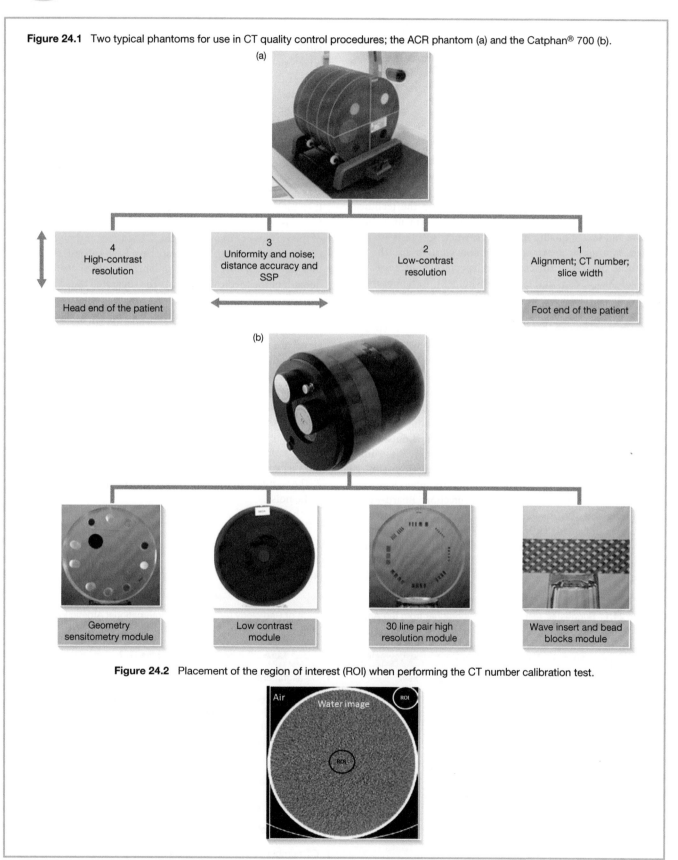

Figure 24.1 Two typical phantoms for use in CT quality control procedures; the ACR phantom (a) and the Catphan® 700 (b).

(a)

| 4 High-contrast resolution | 3 Uniformity and noise; distance accuracy and SSP | 2 Low-contrast resolution | 1 Alignment; CT number; slice width |

Head end of the patient   Foot end of the patient

(b)

| Geometry sensitometry module | Low contrast module | 30 line pair high resolution module | Wave insert and bead blocks module |

Figure 24.2 Placement of the region of interest (ROI) when performing the CT number calibration test.

Air   Water image   ROI

ROI

CT at a Glance, First Edition. Euclid Seeram.

What is quality control?

Quality control (QC) is an essential component of medical imaging and radiation therapy equipment performance. In CT, it consists of a program that periodically tests the CT scanner performance and compares such performance with an established standard. The ultimate purpose of such testing is to ensure that the scanner produces high-quality images with the lowest possible dose to both patients and staff. Such a goal means that QC is a major element of radiation protection optimization in CT, and therefore all CT imaging facilities should have an effective QC program.

Major steps in a QC program

There are at least three important steps in a QC program. These include *acceptance testing*, *routine performance evaluation*, and *error correction*. While the first step involves establishing that the scanner meets the vendor's specifications, the second step is an essential task that deals with monitoring the technical components of the scanner. Such monitoring usually focuses on dose and image quality parameters, where QC tests are performed on a *daily*, *weekly*, *monthly*, and *yearly* basis. The last step in the process, error correction, specifically addresses the results of the QC tests and examines whether the scanner meets what has been referred to as *tolerance limits* or *acceptance limits*. To be an effective and efficient program the QC tests must be carried out on a periodic basis, the results must be interpreted in a prompt manner, and records of these tests must be permanently recorded.

Acceptable or tolerance limits

These are what have been popularly referred to as performance standard ranges of values for a QC test indicating what performance readings are within certain tolerances; if outside this range, the equipment must be serviced immediately. These limits are issued by various authorities such as the American College of Radiology (ACR), the International Atomic Energy Agency (IAEA), the National Radiological Protection Board-Public Health England (NRPB-PHE), and the Radiation Protection Bureau-Health Canada (RPB-HC). For example, while the ACR acceptance limits for the CT number accuracy is set at 0 ± 7 HU (± 5 HU preferred), it is 0 ± 5 for the IAEC; and 0 ± 4 HU for RPB-HC.

Typical phantoms and parameters for QC testing

There are several test tools and phantoms currently available for CT QC, including ones specifically available from CT vendors. Three categories of phantoms are available based on their specific function. These include *image performance phantoms*, *geometric phantoms*, and *quantitative/dosimetry phantoms and instrumentation*. Two such phantoms are illustrated in Figure 24.1, the ACR phantom (Figure 24.1a) and the Catphan® 700 (Figure 24.1b). It is clear that each of these phantoms contains several modules to evaluate specific *image quality parameters*. For example, the ACR phantom has four modules to evaluate high-contrast resolution (spatial resolution); low-contrast resolution; alignment; CT number; slice width; uniformity and noise; distance accuracy; and the slice sensitivity profile.

QC tests

It is not within the scope of this book to describe the numerous QC tests for CT. For example, these tests include *visual inspection* of the various components of the CT scanner and *routine performance* of the scanner. These tests have been categorized as those that can be done by the radiographer and those that are in the domain of the medical physicist. The suggested tests for the radiographer from the ACR and the IAEC are listed in Table 24.1. A few of these include, for example, CT alignment lights; canned projection radiography (SPR) accuracy (also referred to as "scout view," "topogram," "scanogram," or "pilot" – CT vendor terminology; CT number, image noise, image uniformity, and image artifacts; image display and printing; external CT positioning lasers; couch top alignment and positional accuracy; and CT number of multiple materials.

In addition to the above tests, *two routine QC tests* that should be done on a daily basis before scanning patients are:
1 The average CT number for water, also referred to as the CT number calibration.
2 The standard deviation of CT numbers in water. This of course is the noise.

The following is a brief outline of the *CT number calibration* test:
1 Use a water phantom.
2 Scan the phantom with the usual exposure factors and reconstruct the image.

Table 24.1 Suggested tests for the radiographer from the American College of Radiology (ACR) and the International Atomic Energy Agency (IAEA).

Suggested ACR QC tests to be done by the CT technologist:	IAEA QC tests to be done by the CT technologist:
1. CT number for water and standard deviation (noise)	1. CT alignment lights
2. Artifact evaluation	2. Scanned projection radiography (SPR) accuracy, also referred to as "scout view," "topogram," "scanogram," or "pilot" (CT vendor terminology)
3. Display monitor QC	3. CT number, image noise, image uniformity, and image artifacts
4. Visual inspection of certain components of the scanner	4. Image display and printing
	5. External CT positioning lasers
	6. Couch top alignment and positional accuracy
	7. CT number of multiple materials

3 Place the region of interest (ROI) in the center of the image (Figure 24.2) and measure the average CT number.

4 Place the ROI outside the image in a region that is known to be air (Figure 24.2) and check the average CT number for air. It should be −1000 if the scanner is correctly calibrated.

5 The acceptance limits should be based on the authority providing recommendations in the specific country. For example it is 0 ± 5 for the IAEC.

The *standard deviation of the CT number* test involves the following:

1 Use the same image as in Test 1.

2 Place the ROI near the center of the image and measure the standard deviation of the CT number (see Figure 19.2). This value should be very small.

3 The actual acceptance limits must be determined by examination of past measurements that were presumably performed when the performance of the CT scanner was good. The technique must stay the same for this measurement from day to day. If the standard deviation starts to increase, this indicates a "noisier" image with more variation in pixel-to-pixel CT numbers and poorer low-contrast resolution.

Index

CT at a Glance, First Edition. Euclid Seeram.
© 2018 John Wiley & Sons, Ltd. Published 2018 by John Wiley & Sons, Ltd.